Telecourse Guide

for

Psychology
The Study of Human Behavior
Fifth Edition

Michael S. Werthman

for

Coast Community College District
Costa Mesa, California

Coast Community College District

William M. Vega, Chancellor, Coast Community College District

Leslie N. Purdy, President, Coastline Community College

Dan C. Jones, Administrative Dean, Instructional Systems Development

Judy Garvey, Publications Supervisor

Wendy Sacket, Senior Publications Assistant

Thien Vu, Publications Assistant

The Telecourse *Psychology: The Study of Human Behavior* is produced by the Coast Community College District in cooperation with the INTELECOM (the Southern California Consortium for Community College Television); the Northern Illinois Learning Resources Cooperative; the State of Florida Department of Education; the Dallas County Community College District; the Higher Education Telecommunications Association of Oklahoma; TVOntario; and Prentice Hall.

ISBN 0-321-05957-3

Preface

To the Student

Welcome to *Psychology: The Study of Human Behavior*, a telecourse in introductory psychology. Whether you are planning a career in psychology or taking the course to gain personal insights about yourself and others, we hope that you will find this a useful and interesting course of study.

This telecourse is designed to cover the concepts, vocabulary, and subjects usually treated in an on-campus college introductory psychology course typical of any two- or four-year college or university. As with a campus course, this telecourse has a text, a student study guide, tests, and assignments. But, unlike a campus course, this telecourse also includes 26 half-hour video programs. The text is *Psychology*, sixth edition, by Carole Wade and Carol Tavris (Prentice Hall, 2000). This book, *Telecourse Guide for Psychology: The Study of Human Behavior*, will direct your study throughout the course, providing reading and viewing assignments, study activities, and practice test questions. Note that each chapter of this guide begins with a list of the assignments to make it easier for you to plan your studies. Just inside the back cover is a Quick Reference Guide that shows how each chapter in this book relates to the corresponding Wade and Tavris text reading assignment and video program.

One of the features of this course is its emphasis on critical thinking. The text, video programs, and this telecourse guide will help you improve your ability to use critical thinking to facilitate learning and improve your everyday living. Information and exercises in the course encourage you to approach new material analytically and evaluate all data and ideas critically. Through the use of your ever-improving critical thinking skills, you will find it easier to learn and remember even the most complex concepts.

Course Goals

The designers, academic advisors, and producers of this telecourse have defined the major goals to be achieved by students taking *Psychology: The Study of Human Behavior*. These goals include cognitive goals (academic or intellectual objectives) and affective goals (personal goals involving your feelings and behavior).

Cognitive Goals

By the end of the course, we want you to be able to:

1. Define psychology and explain how the focus of psychology is different from that of other social and biological sciences.

2. Describe the major features of the scientific method and explain the steps and key considerations in research.

3. Define basic psychological terminology and explain important features of major psychological concepts and theories.

4. Identify leading contributors to the field of psychology and describe their work.

5. Explain how biological, psychological, and social factors can affect behavior.

6. Identify and describe specific psychological principles in real-life situations.

7. Critically analyze information about human behavior and distinguish between conclusions supported by scientific evidence and conclusions based on nonscientific ways of knowing.

8. Recognize real-life situations that may call for professional psychological help and know how to use community resources to find help when needed.

Affective Goals

By the end of the course, we want you to be able to:

1. Develop a positive attitude toward the discipline of psychology.

2. Appreciate how psychology can enrich and help to explain individual experience and social interaction.

3. Appreciate similarities and differences between individuals.

4. Appreciate how culture, gender, and other group identities can influence self-awareness and interactions between people.

5. Appreciate the impact of prejudices on attitudes and behaviors.

6. Appreciate that various information sources differ as to quality and reliability.

7. Appreciate that our understanding of human behavior has evolved and changed over the years and that increasingly refined psychological theories have been developed.

How to Take a Telecourse

- Buy the text and telecourse study guide. Do not try to get through the course without these books. Watch each of the video programs, because they do not merely repeat information provided in the books. You will need to read and study the text and view the programs in order to pass the examinations. Use the Quick Reference Guide printed inside the back cover of this book to keep track of your reading assignments and the times when the video programs will be broadcast (the guide has spaces for you to fill in when each program may be viewed in your area).

- Keep up with your work for this course every week. Even if you do not have any class sessions on campus or any assignments to turn in, it is very important to read the text and do the assignments in the study guide at about the same time that you watch the programs every week. The programs will make more sense to you if you follow the study sequence outlined in each chapter of this study guide and do some reading before viewing the programs. But, most important, try to keep up with your work; do not fall behind, even a week or two. Students taking telecourses find that it is difficult to catch up after missing the course work presented over a period of two weeks or longer. Set aside viewing, reading, and study time every week and stick to your schedule.

- Get in touch with the faculty member for this course at your college or university. He or she can answer any questions you have about the course content, help you catch up if you are behind, advise you about additional assignments, discuss the types of test questions that will be used, or tell you where you may be able to watch the programs should you happen to miss a broadcast. The instructor wants to hear from you to find out what you think of the course; institutions often experiment with distance-learning courses and instructors are concerned to hear how students like the programs, the tests, and other aspects of the course. So don't hesitate to call, write, or visit your instructor.

- Follow the activities listed in each study guide chapter. Each chapter has been written to help you. Reading the study guide chapter will often provide you with the information you would get in a classroom if you were taking the course on campus. You will find out what to watch for in the programs and what pages to read in the textbook (Assignments), what topics covered in the lesson are the major ones, and what particular terms and concepts you should know. Each chapter has a section in which you can review the material (Review Exercises, with matching, completion, true-false, and short-answer exercises) and a multiple-choice Self-Test that you should use to see if you have mastered the information. Answers to the test items are given and text pages are referenced so that you can check yourself and review the material if necessary. There are also intriguing Study Activities, for which your instructor may decide to award extra credit.

- Read the summaries at the end of each chapter in your text. A review of the summary will not substitute for careful study of the assignment as a whole, but you should study the summary carefully after reading the chapter, and at other times as you study the lesson, to aid your recall of important information.

- Watch the programs without interruption or distraction. Tell your family or friends that you are working on a course assignment and should not be disturbed. Each program is only thirty minutes long and, if your viewing is interrupted or you cannot concentrate, you may lose the point or miss a critical scene. We do not recommend taking detailed notes during a program, but if you want to have a pad of paper and a pencil on hand, writing down a few key terms may help you remember crucial ideas. Take a few minutes after the program and try to summarize what you have seen, especially the important concepts covered. Some students rent videotapes or make videotapes or audiotapes of programs for their personal use in reviewing and studying the material.

- If you do miss a program or fall behind, don't give up. Many television stations and cable companies provide repeats of the programs later in the week or on weekends. Most colleges have cassette copies of the program available in libraries or media centers where you can go and review any you have missed. Call on your course faculty member or manager to help you if you have problems of any kind. The faculty person is assigned specifically to help you.

Acknowledgments

The telecourse *Psychology: The Study of Human Behavior* is the result of many months of work by many individuals. Production of the video programs, the textbook, the telecourse guide, and related test materials took more than two years.

The following are some of the individuals who contributed in creating this telecourse:

Members of the Telecourse Advisory Committee:

Frank Bagrash, Ph.D., California State University, Fullerton

Ted Barnes, Coastline Community College

Horace Black, Golden West College

Gerald E. Burson, Ed.D., Navarro College

Michael Catchpole, Ph.D., North Island College

Ethel McClatchey, Los Angeles Community College District

Barbara Hildebrand, Lincoln Land Community College

George Mount, Ph.D., Dallas County Community College

Sheryl S. Peterson, St. Petersburg Junior College

Special Academic Advisors:

Carol Tavris, Ph.D.

Carole Wade, Ph.D., Dominican College of San Rafael

Television production team:

David Stone, Harry Ratner, Eve Coté, Laurie Harer, Marjorie Kustra, Ted Boehler, Dorothy McCollom, and the many writers, editors, camera operators, and researchers who made the programs.

In addition, special thanks are extended to Joann Jelly, Ph.D., instructor of psychology at Barstow College (California), who reviewed the content and accuracy of this fifth edition of the telecourse student guide. Additional thanks are extended to Cyndy Taylor and to Bill Webber and his staff at Prentice Hall.

Contents

Lesson 1

What Is Psychology?

Assignments

For the most systematic coverage of this lesson, we suggest that you complete the assignments in the sequence listed below.

Before viewing the video program:

- Read the "Learning Objectives" and "Overview" for this lesson. Use the Learning Objectives to guide your reading, viewing, and thinking.

- Read the "Viewing Notes" for this lesson.

- Read Chapter 1, "The Science of Psychology?," in the Wade and Tavris text. First, familiarize yourself with its contents by reading the Chapter Outline. As you read, note terms and concepts set in bold or italic type, especially those defined in the margins. Take the Quick Quizzes to check your understanding of material being described and explained.

View the video program, "What Is Psychology?"

After viewing the video program:

- Briefly note your answers to the questions at the end of the "Viewing Notes."

- Review all reading assignments for this lesson, including the Summary at the end of Chapter 1 in the textbook.

- Complete the "Review Exercises" to strengthen your understanding of this lesson's central concepts and terminology. Pay special attention to the "Vocabulary Check" exercise and the additional terms and concepts that follow—page references indicate where in the text assignment each term is defined. [Remember: there is a complete Glossary at the end of the text.]

- Take the "Self-Test" to measure the degree to which you are achieving this lesson's learning objectives. Check your answers against the "Answer Key" and review when necessary.

- Follow the suggestions in the "Study Activities" section at the end of this lesson and complete any other activities and projects assigned by your instructor.

Learning Objectives

When you have completed all assignments in this lesson, you should be able to:

1. Define psychology, and explain psychology's goal: to describe, understand, predict, and modify or control behavior and mental processes.

2. Identify and explain at least one example of psychological research findings that contradict or significantly amplify a popular commonsense explanation of human behavior.

3. Describe the basic approach of each major perspective in psychology—biological (or physiological), learning (or behavioral), cognitive, psychodynamic (including psychoanalytic and other clinical approaches), and sociocultural—and discuss the use of integrated or eclectic approaches.

4. Distinguish between basic and applied psychology, and describe the various types of work done by psychologists in society.

5. List the eight rules essential to thinking critically and creatively about psychology.

Overview

Whether or not you are really interested in psychology, psychology is interested in you. In fact, you are what psychologists study. You, the individual and the member of groups, the ordinary person or the exceptional one. Whether you are stable and satisfied or disturbed and unhappy, psychology is interested in how you behave, how you think, what you feel. As you increase your knowledge of what psychology is and what psychologists do, you will begin to appreciate that the more you know about this fascinating subject, the more you know yourself and the people with whom you share this world. This first lesson in the telecourse *Psychology: The Study of Human Behavior* introduces you to the field and should pique your interest in the topics covered in the other lessons.

This lesson clearly defines **psychology** and identifies its chief goals. It shows how psychology's rigorous and systematic procedures differentiate it from common sense and various other nonscientific approaches to understanding human experience. After briefly tracing the origins of psychology, the lesson describes the major perspectives in psychology: **biological** (or **physiological**), **learning** (or **behavioral**), **cognitive**, **psychodynamic** (including **psychoanalytic** and other clinical approaches), and **sociocultural**. It also discusses the use of integrated, or **eclectic**, approaches.

The lesson explains the differences between **basic** and **applied** psychology. It enumerates the many divisions, or specialties, within psychology and describes the various types of work done by psychologists.

The essential rules of **critical thinking** are presented in this lesson, giving readers a foundation of understanding upon which to base analyses of problems throughout the course.

The video program and text assignment introduce many of the topics covered in depth in other lessons. This lesson previews such important subjects as personality and interpersonal relationships; the functions of sleep; the role of language; the nature of perception, memory, emotion, and intelligence; the biological (genetic) and environmental (sociocultural) bases of behavior; and the origins of human wisdom and folly.

The video program "What Is Psychology?" deals with the nature of psychology and what its practitioners do. Experts in the field discuss their work, which seeks to describe, understand, predict, and control or modify the seemingly bewildering variety of human behavior. They assert that, despite the great diversity of humanity, psychology undertakes to explain individual human behavior and mental processes.

As you watch the video program, consider the following questions:

1. What does the behavior of such diverse individuals as serial killers and selfless people who help the poor and the desperate tell psychologists about the range of human motivations?

2. What can knowledge of tribal societies, ancient cultures, and religious traditions contribute to modern psychologists' attainment of meaningful insights?

3. What role did concepts such as the four humors, phrenology, and mesmerism play in the development of a true science of psychology?

4. What distinguishes psychology from other disciplines and approaches to explaining human behavior?

5. What are the major approaches or perspectives in modern psychology?

6. As discussed by Michael Mahoney, what are the "five families" of the clinical approach to psychology, which are further subdivided into the more than 300 forms of psychotherapy currently being practiced?

7. What are some of the principal subjects that are of interest to psychologists and that are covered in this course?

Review Exercises

Vocabulary Check

Match the following key terms and concepts with the appropriate definitions from the list below.

1. _L_ applied psychology (p. 23)

2. _H_ behaviorism (p. 18; video)

3. _A_ biological (or physiological) perspective (p. 18; video)

4. _J_ cognitive perspective (p. 18; video)

5. _G_ critical thinking (p. 5)

6. _B_ eclectic (page 27; video)

7. _I_ empirical (p. 2)

8. _C_ functionalism (p. 16)

9. _M_ humanist psychology (humanism) (p. 19)

10. _F_ psychology (p. 2; video)

11. _D_ social-cognitive learning theory (p. 18)

12. _E_ sociocultural perspective (p. 18)

13. _K_ structuralism (p. 15)

a. emphasizes bodily events and changes associated with feelings, actions, and thoughts

b. using the best features of diverse theories and schools of thought

c. an early approach to psychology that stressed the function or purpose of behavior and consciousness

d. the theory that human social behavior is learned through observation and imitation of others, positive consequences, and cognitive processes such as plans and expectations

e. emphasizes social and cultural influences on behavior

f. the scientific study of behavior and mental processes and how they are affected by an organism's physical state, mental state, and external environment

g. the ability and willingness to assess claims and make objective judgments on the basis of well-supported reasons

h. emphasizes the study of objectively observable behavior rather than inner mental experiences and stresses the role of the environment as a determinant of human and animal behavior

i. relying on or derived from observation, experimentation, or measurement

j.   emphasizes mental processes in perception, memory, language, problem solving, and other areas of behavior

k.   an early approach to psychology that stressed analysis of immediate experience (sensations, images, feelings) into basic elements

l.   the study of psychological issues that have direct practical significance and the application of psychological findings

m.   emphasizes personal growth and the achievement of human potential more than it does the scientific

Other Key Terms and Concepts

basic psychology (p. 23)

cultural psychologists (p. 19)

evolutionary psychology (p. 18)

feminist psychology (p. 20)

learning perspective (p. 18)

psychiatry (p. 25)

psychoanalysis (p. 16; video)

psychodynamic perspective (p. 19)

psychotherapy (p. 24; video)

social psychology (video)

trained introspection (video)

Completion

Fill each blank with the most appropriate term from the list of answers below.

14.   Psychology's goals are to _____, _____, _____, and _____ behavior and mental processes.

15.   Because _____ is full of contradictions and tends to oversimplify, it can be used to support two sides of an argument.

16.   One of psychology's sister sciences is _____, which is devoted to the medical study, diagnosis, treatment, and prevention of mental disorders.

17.   The two names most often associated with behaviorism are _____ and _____.

18.   _____ is usually associated with psychoanalysis.

19.   Psychologists who seek knowledge for its own sake work in the discipline known as _____, whereas psychologists who are largely concerned with the practical uses of knowledge work in a field known as _____.

20. There are many specialties within psychology, including _____ psychology, which deals with how groups, institutions, and the social context influence individuals and vice versa, and _____ psychology, which is devoted to the study of such behavior in the workplace as decision making, morale, motivation, and productivity.

21. _____ psychologists have spurred the growth of research on topics such as menstruation, motherhood, the dynamics of power in close relationships, and changing definitions of masculinity and femininity.

22. Critical thinking is the ability to look for flaws in arguments and resist claims that have no supporting evidence, and such thinking should be _____ and _____, not merely negative thinking.

anthropology	describe	predict
applied psychology	feminist	psychiatry
basic psychology	industrial/	Sigmund Freud
B. F. Skinner	organizational	social
common sense	John B. Watson	social or behavioral
constructive	modify or control	sociology
creative	phrenology	understand

True-False

Read the following statements carefully and mark each true (T) or false (F).

23. ___ Psychology is the scientific study of human behavior, with little concern for people's physical or mental states.

24. ___ Psychology makes no effort to predict behavior or mental processes.

25. ___ Unlike people who rely on little more than common sense to form opinions about human behavior and experience, psychologists must follow rigorous and systematic procedures.

26. ___ The findings of psychological research seldom, if ever, confirm commonsense opinions about human nature.

27. ___ Psychiatry is the medical study, diagnosis, treatment, and prevention of mental disorders.

28. ___ The learning (or behavioral) and humanistic perspectives approach psychology in largely the same ways.

29. ___ Cognitive psychology doesn't have a unifying theory or any one acknowledged spokesperson.

30. ___ Basic psychology is essentially "pure" research that may or may not have apparent practical application.

31. ___ Because there are few nonclinical specialties in psychology, most psychologists either do basic research or work with individuals who have emotional problems.

32. ___ Critical thinking is basically negative thinking.

33. ___ Being able to think critically involves learning to live with uncertainty, to accept that in some cases there is no evidence on which to base a certain conclusion.

Short-Answer Questions

As a final review exercise, write brief answers to demonstrate that you are achieving the learning objectives of this lesson.

1. Define psychology, and explain psychology's goal: to describe, understand, predict, and modify or control behavior and mental processes.

2. Identify and explain at least one example of psychological research findings that contradict or significantly amplify a popular commonsense explanation of human behavior.

3. Describe the basic approach of each major perspective in psychology—biological (or physiological), learning (or behavioral), cognitive, psychodynamic (including psychoanalytic and other clinical approaches), and sociocultural—and discuss the use of integrated or eclectic approaches.

4. Distinguish between basic and applied psychology, and describe the various types of work done by psychologists in society.

5. List the eight rules essential to thinking critically and creatively about psychology.

Self-Test

1. Psychology may best be described as the scientific study of
   _____ and _____.
   a. mental states; physical states
   b. thoughts; emotions
   c. behavior; mental processes
   d. mental health; mental illness

2. Psychologists usually consider psychology, as a formal science, to
   have begun in the _____ century.
   a. eighteenth
   b. early nineteenth
   c. late nineteenth
   d. early twentieth

3. Which of the following is **NOT** one of psychology's goals?
   a. understanding behavior and mental processes
   b. approving behavior and mental processes
   c. predicting behavior and mental processes
   d. controlling or modifying behavior and mental processes

4. Whereas the _____ asked what happens when an organism does
   something, the _____ asked how and why.
   a. functionalists; behaviorists
   b. structuralists; introspectionists
   c. functionalists; structuralists
   d. structuralists; functionalists

5. Psychological research on a given topic
   a. nearly always contradicts commonsense opinions.
   b. usually confirms commonsense opinions.
   c. almost never confirms commonsense opinions.
   d. may or may not confirm commonsense opinions.

6. Some proponents of the learning perspective have suggested that if psychology were ever to be objective and scientific, it would have to give up its preoccupation with
   a. abnormal behavior and mental illness.
   b. emphasis on unconscious forces.
   c. the physiology of behavior.
   d. self-realization and human potential.

7. _____ psychologists are particularly interested in helping people express themselves creatively and achieve their full human potential.
   a. Behavioral
   b. Gestalt
   c. Humanist
   d. Physiological

8. _____ is identified with the beginning of physiological (biological) psychology.
   a. William B. Watson
   b. Wilhelm Wundt
   c. Abraham Maslow
   d. Sigmund Freud

9. _____ psychologists maintain that a pervasive bias in research exists and that if psychology is to become more socially useful, such biases must be corrected.
   a. Feminist
   b. Cognitive
   c. Physiological
   d. Behavioral

10. _____ psychologists draw upon what they believe to be the best features of diverse theories and schools of thought.

   a. Holistic

   b. Humanistic

   c. Eclectic

   d. Cognitive

11. Which of the following would be of greatest interest to someone working in basic psychology?

   a. counseling the emotionally disturbed

   b. performing polygraph (lie detector) tests on individuals suspected of crimes

   c. preventing child abuse

   d. determining the causes of shyness

12. Which of the following would be **LEAST** likely to practice psychotherapy?

   a. clinical psychologists

   b. psychometric psychologists

   c. psychiatrists

   d. psychoanalysts

13. _____ is the medical specialty concerned with mental disorders, maladjustment, and abnormal behavior, in which treatment is provided by practitioners with medical degrees.

   a. Clinical psychology

   b. Social psychology

   c. Psychiatry

   d. Psychoanalysis

14. More than two-thirds of new psychology doctorates go to practitioners, whose object is to

   a. teach psychology in high schools and colleges.

   b. do pure, basic research.

   c. understand and improve physical and mental health.

   d. design and evaluate tests of mental abilities.

15. One of the values of critical thinking is that it fosters the ability to be
    _____ and _____.

    a. creative; constructive

    b. ambitious; efficient

    c. observant; self-conscious

    d. confident; opinionated

16. Which of the following can undermine critical thinking?

    a. asking too many questions

    b. reasoning emotionally

    c. considering other interpretations

    d. tolerating uncertainty

17. Which of the following is **NOT** true of critical thinkers?

    a. They examine evidence.

    b. They are aware of their own assumptions and are willing to
       question them.

    c. They accept the value of easy generalizations.

    d. They define their terms.

Study Activities

The following activity challenges you to use your critical thinking and demonstrate how what you are learning can be applied to you and your own life. Try this activity and/or those your instructor assigns.

In the Wade and Tavris textbook, review pages 22–26 about what psychologists do. With that information fresh in your mind, begin an "Experiences with Psychology" memoir listing what you know about the interests, activities, and contributions of psychologists. Add to your memoir throughout this course.

You might start with any personal experiences you have had with psychology and psychologists. In some cases you may not have realized that certain people you encountered were trained in psychology. For example, have you ever taken an aptitude test, placement test, or personality profile? If so, list the details of such experiences in your memoir. Indicate when and under what circumstances the events you are recording took place. Try to be as detailed as possible; it will make your document more useful and will give you training in being specific and thorough. Record other personal experiences, perhaps with a school psychologist, a family counselor, even a therapist. [Any information you consider sufficiently personal—or embarrassing—need not be made a part of a document intended to be read by others. Write everything down, but keep highly confidential material separate, for your own use only.]

You can also compile information from the media: newspapers, magazines, books, films, and television. Don't exclude fictionalized accounts of psychology and psychologists. Such pop cultural depictions can reveal a great deal about how psychology is regarded in our society.

Anything you read or hear about psychology can be added to your memoir. Look for reports of psychology research, new forms of therapy, or the role psychologists may have played in some public event. And you can, of course, read psychology journal articles and report on what you learn. You may also want to review pages 28–29 in the Wade and Tavris textbook on what psychology can and can't do for you. This section should give you additional ideas about what psychologists do and sharpen your awareness of the sorts of activities in which they may be involved. The whole point is to record what you are learning about psychology as a science and about the many ways in which it touches the problems and activities of people and institutions of all kinds.

How Psychologists Know What They Know

Assignments

For the most systematic coverage of this lesson, we suggest that you complete the assignments in the sequence listed below.

Before viewing the video program:

- Read the "Learning Objectives" and "Overview" for this lesson. Use the Learning Objectives to guide your reading, viewing, and thinking.

- Read the "Viewing Notes" for this lesson.

- Read Chapter 2, "How Psychologists Do Research," in the Wade and Tavris text. First, familiarize yourself with its contents by reading the Chapter Outline. As you read, note terms and concepts set in bold or italic type, especially those defined in the margins. Take the Quick Quizzes to check your understanding of material being described and explained.

View the video program, "Research Methods"

After viewing the video program:

- Briefly note your answers to the questions at the end of the "Viewing Notes."

- Review all reading assignments for this lesson, including the Summary at the end of Chapter 2 in the textbook.

- Complete the "Review Exercises" to strengthen your understanding of this lesson's central concepts and terminology. Pay special attention to the "Vocabulary Check" exercise and the additional terms and concepts that follow—page references indicate where in the text assignment each term is defined. [Remember: there is a complete Glossary at the end of the text.]

- Take the "Self-Test" to measure the degree to which you are achieving this lesson's learning objectives. Check your answers against the "Answer Key" and review when necessary.

- Follow the suggestions in the "Study Activities" section at the end of this lesson and complete any other activities and projects assigned by your instructor.

Learning Objectives

When you have completed all assignments in this lesson, you should be able to:

1. Identify and explain features that distinguish scientific from nonscientific ways of knowing. Discuss reasons why using sound scientific methodology is important.

2. Describe the following descriptive methods of research: case studies, naturalistic observation, laboratory observation, surveys, and tests.

3. Explain correlational research and why findings from correlational studies must be interpreted cautiously.

4. Distinguish between the goal of descriptive research methods and the goal of "the experiment."

5. Define the following terms and identify examples in given research experiments or an experiment of your own design: independent variable, dependent variable, control group, experimental group, double-blind study.

6. Discuss several possible problems involved in interpreting research findings.

7. Discuss ethical issues psychologists need to consider in designing and performing research experiments.

Overview

A bad study, even if it is repeated a hundred times, can tell us nothing. As textbook authors Wade and Tavris put it: "If the assumptions and methods of a study are faulty, so are the results and conclusions based on them. Ultimately, what we know about human behavior is inseparable from how we know it." This lesson provides factual support for these contentions, emphasizing that psychological research conducted without sound scientific methodology is of little or no value—and, as the video program makes unmistakably clear, can even be harmful.

This lesson alerts students to the differences between science and pseudoscience, between scientific and nonscientific ways of knowing. It explains what makes research scientific, identifying such key factors as skepticism, reliance on empirical evidence, precision, openness, and willingness to make "risky predictions," to adhere to the **principle of falsifiability**. It defines such central concepts as **hypothesis**, **theory**, **operational definition**, and **replication**.

Several descriptive methods of research—**case studies** (**case histories**), **naturalistic observation** and **laboratory observation**, **surveys**, and **tests**—are introduced. **Sampling** (including the importance of **representative sampling**) is described, and the value and limitations of **correlational studies** (descriptive research that quantifies the relationship between two or more variables) are pointed out.

This lesson explains that descriptive research and experiments have different goals. It defines the basic terminology of experimental research: **variables**, **control groups** and **experimental groups**, **random assignment**, **single-blind** and **double-blind studies**, **experimenter effects**, and **placebos**.

The video program and text focus on the application of research findings to practical, real-world needs and problems. Among the examples of the positive impact of psychological research is the video account of the development of cognitive interview techniques to replace the far less effective traditional police interviews. The lesson also highlights the negative impact of research that employs less-than-rigorous scientific methods. It also asks students to consider such difficult ethical issues as the use of animals in research and researchers' use of deception in dealing with human subjects.

Viewing Notes

The video program "Research Methods" contains several vivid examples of the importance of using sound scientific methodology and of the impact of psychological research on ordinary people in real-world situations. The initial episode in the video includes old film footage showing a lobotomy, a form of psychosurgery performed on some 50,000 mental patients in the United States from the late 1930s to mid-1950s. Ancient—even prehistoric—healers appear to have performed a sort of surgery (called trepanning) that involved opening the skull. Lobotomies are now seldom performed, having been shown to be unduly damaging to patients. Other forms of psychosurgery are still performed, and although they are more refined and are evaluated more scientifically than lobotomies were, psychosurgery itself remains highly controversial.

This video lesson contains an equally provocative episode on autism. It explains how an influential theory of that mysterious childhood ailment had a tragic impact on many individuals' lives until rigorous scientific investigation showed the theory to be erroneous. There is also an exciting and encouraging segment on the so-called cognitive interview technique being adopted by police investigators. It demonstrates how scientifically sound psychological research can be employed to help solve serious everyday problems.

As you watch the video program, consider the following questions:

1. What factors led most clinicians to reject lobotomies as a viable treatment option?

2. How and to whom was the erroneous, scientifically unsound hypothesis about the causes of autism harmful?

3. What research methods and evidence contributed to the creation of a scientifically rigorous theory to replace the insufficiently supported speculations on the causes of autism?

4. What are the principal differences between the methods used in a standard police interview and the techniques of a cognitive interview?

5. What are some of the examples in this video program that support Irv Maltzman's contention that we all must be skeptical, must question, must doubt even purported authorities and famous experts, and must recognize that our ultimate safeguard against misinformation and unsupported theories is our own intelligence?

Review Exercises

Vocabulary Check

Match the following key terms and concepts with the appropriate definitions from the list below.

1. _G_ case study (case history) (p. 38; video)

2. _M_ control group (p. 50)

3. _O_ correlation (p. 44)

4. _D_ double-blind study (p. 51)

5. _I_ experiment (p. 48)

6. _F_ hypothesis (p. 34; video)

7. _A_ longitudinal study (p. 57)

8. _K_ norms (in testing) (p. 41)

9. _N_ principle of falsifiability (p. 35)

10. _B_ reliable test (p. 41)

11. _E_ representative sample (p. 43)

12. _L_ surveys (p. 43)

13. _J_ theory (p. 34)

14. _H_ valid test (p. 42)

15. _C_ variables (p. 44)

a. a study in which subjects are followed and periodically reassessed over a long period of time

b. a test that yields consistent scores from one time and place to another   *reliable*

c. characteristics of behavior or experience that can be measured or described and manipulated and assessed in scientific studies   *variables*

d. an experiment in which neither the subjects nor the researchers know which subjects are in the control group(s) and which are in the experimental group(s) until after the results are tallied

e. a group of subjects for study who are selected from a given population and reflect its characteristics   *representative*

f. a statement that attempts to predict or account for a set of phenomena   *hypothesis*

g. a detailed description of a particular individual who is being studied or receiving treatment

h. a test that measures what it was designed to measure

i. a controlled test of hypotheses in which the researcher manipulates one or more variables to discover the resulting effect on others, while holding other conditions constant

j. an organized system of assumptions and principles that claims to explain a specified set of phenomena and their interrelationships

k. in test construction, established standards of performance

l. questionnaires and interviews that ask people about their experiences, attitudes, or opinions

m. a comparison group of subjects who are not exposed to the same "treatment" or manipulation of the independent variable as experimental subjects are

n. holds each scientist to stating an idea in such a way that it can be refuted, or disproved by counterevidence

o. a measure of how strongly two or more variables are related to one another

Other Key Terms and Concepts

arithmetic mean (p. 55)

coefficient of correlation (p. 46)

control condition (p. 50)

correlational study (p. 44)

cross-sectional study (p. 57)

dependent variable (p. 48)

descriptive methods (p. 38)

descriptive statistics (p. 55)

experimental group (p. 50)

experimenter effects (p. 50)

field research (p. 52)

independent variable (p. 48)

inferential statistics (p. 55)

informed consent (p. 59)

laboratory observation (p. 40)

meta-analysis (p. 57)

naturalistic observation (p. 39)

negative correlation (p. 45)

observational study (p. 39)

operational definition (p. 35)

placebo (p. 50)

population (p. 43)

positive correlation (p. 45)

psychological tests (p. 41)

random assignment (p. 50)

replicate (p. 35)

sample (p. 43)

significance tests (p. 55)

single-blind study (p. 50)

standardize (p. 41)

volunteer bias (p. 43)

Completion

Fill each blank with the most appropriate term from the list of answers below.

16. All people are vulnerable to the _confirmation bias_, the tendency to look for evidence that supports their ideas and to ignore evidence that does not.

17. Key features that distinguish a scientist from someone who employs nonscientific ways of knowing are _presicion_, _openess_, _skeptism_, _reliance of empiric_, and _willingness to make risky predictions_.

18. When ethologists study the behavior of apes in the wild, they are employing _naturalistic_, but when the same or similar animals are studied in an environment created and controlled by scientists, those apes are subjected to _laboratory_ observation.

19. The _population_ is the entire set of individuals from which a sample is drawn.

20. Various types of _psychological_ tests can be used to measure personality traits, emotional states, aptitudes, interests, abilities, and values.

21. Correlational studies can be misleading, because no matter how strong a correlation may be demonstrated between two or more variables, a correlation does not show _causation_.

22. Unlike descriptive studies, a psychological experiment allows the researcher to _control_ the situation being studied and is intended to explain the _causes_ of behavior.

23. The aspect of an experiment manipulated by the researcher is called the _independent_; the reaction of the subjects, which the researcher tries to predict, is known as the _dependent_.

24. Unintended changes in subjects' behavior due to inadvertent cues from the researcher are called _experimenter effects_.

25. The major difficulty in interpreting _laboratory_ experiments is that they may not generalize well to the real world.

26. One of the uses of _meta-analysis_ is to statistically combine the results of many studies to help researchers better understand a topic and relate their findings to the real world, instead of merely assessing the results of each study separately.

27. The American Psychological Association (APA) has a formal code and there are federal regulations that attempt to prevent or lessen _ethical_ problems in both clinical practice and psychological research.

causation

causes

confirmation bias

control

dependent variable

ethical

experimenter
    effects

independent variable

laboratory

laboratory observation

meta-analysis

naturalistic
    observation

openness

population

precision

psychological

reliance on empirical
    evidence

skepticism

willingness to make
    "risky
    predictions"

True-False

Read the following statements carefully and mark each true (T) or false (F).

28. _F_ Scientists are as likely as nonscientists to look for evidence that supports their ideas and to ignore evidence that doesn't.

29. _T_ Any theory that cannot in principle be refuted is unscientific.

30. _F_ A case study (or case history) is a research method for describing the behavior of a large group of subjects.

31. _T_ Jane Goodall's studies of chimps in the wild exemplify naturalistic observation.

32. _F_ Surveys are an effective and popular form of information gathering because they invariably examine representative samples of the entire population the researchers wish to describe.

33. _T_ A correlation is a numerical measure of the strength of a relationship between two or more things.

34. _T_ Descriptive psychological research may lead researchers to propose explanations of behavior, but it usually requires experimentation to identify causes.

35. _F_ In research studying the possible effects of a drug, members of a control group will receive that substance, while the experimental group will be given a placebo.

36. _F_ Single-blind studies take half as long as double-blind experiments.

37. _T_ The findings from cross-sectional and longitudinal studies of mental abilities may conflict.

38. _F_ The often bitter controversy over the ethics of using animals in medical research has not been extended to include psychological studies involving rats, pigeons, and other species.

Short-Answer Questions

As a final review exercise, write brief answers to demonstrate that you are achieving the learning objectives of this lesson.

1. Identify and explain features that distinguish scientific from nonscientific ways of knowing. Discuss reasons why using sound scientific methodology is important.

2. Describe the following descriptive methods of research: case studies, naturalistic observation, laboratory observation, surveys, and tests.

3. Explain correlational research and why findings from correlational studies must be interpreted cautiously.

4. Distinguish between the goal of descriptive research methods and the goal of "the experiment."

5. Define the following terms and identify examples in given research experiments or an experiment of your own design: independent variable, dependent variable, control group, experimental group, double-blind study.

6. Discuss several possible problems involved in interpreting research findings.

7. Discuss ethical issues psychologists need to consider in designing and performing research experiments.

Self-Test

1. Scientific research methods are

   a. only applied to psychological problems by scientists who are not themselves psychologists.

   b. no more precise or dependable than nonscientific ways of knowing.

   (c.) the tools of the psychologist's trade.

   d. of limited utility in the real world.

2. Despite Bruno Bettelheim's reputation for important work as a psychoanalyst, his influential notions about the causes of autism were proved to be harmfully incorrect because he

   a. concentrated on children with autism without taking the parents of such children into account.

   b. failed to employ sound scientific methodology before publishing his conclusions.

   c. neglected to use MRI and PET scans to check his conclusions.

   d. did not know what most other authorities already believed.

3. Which of the following is **NOT** one of the key characteristics of an ideal scientist (one who rigorously employs sound scientific methodology)?

   a. reliance on empirical evidence

   (b.) unwillingness to make "risky predictions"

   c. skepticism

   d. precision

4. Which sort of theory is most likely to be unscientific?

   a. one that is an organized system of assumptions and principles

   b. one that has come to be accepted by a large part of the scientific community and is consistent with many different observations and inconsistent with only a few

   c. one that purports to explain everything that could possibly happen

   (d.) one that purports to explain certain phenomena

5. If you were studying the personality and behavior of a particular individual, which of these descriptive methods of research would probably be the best to employ?

   a. laboratory observation

   b. naturalistic observation

   c. case history

   d. survey

6. If you were studying the behavior of spectators at sporting events, which of these descriptive methods of research would probably be the best to employ?

   a. laboratory observation

   b. naturalistic observation

   c. case history

   d. survey

7. The findings of informal surveys that invite people to register their opinions by calling or writing in are often untrustworthy because

   a. of volunteer bias.

   b. the sample is usually too small.

   c. some people contribute more than one opinion.

   d. people always lie when responding to surveys.

8. Scientists refer to a test that yields the same results from one time and place to another as

   a. reliable.

   b. valid.

   c. consistent.

   d. predictable.

9. When high values of one variable are associated with high values of another variable, or low values are similarly associated with low values, there is a

a. positive correlation.

b. negative correlation.

c. dependent variable.

d. coefficient of correlation.

10. The statistic used to express a correlation is called the

a. positive correlation.

b. negative correlation.

c. dependent variable.

d. coefficient of correlation.

11. Correlational studies can be misleading because they

a. usually show only positive correlations.

b. usually show only negative correlations.

c. do not show causation.

d. do not employ scientific methodology.

12. Unlike a psychological study using descriptive methods, an experiment permits the researcher to _Control_ the situation being studied.

a. choose

b. control

c. analyze

d. observe

13. Which of the following research methods is most likely to help explain the cause of individual or group behavior?

a. surveys

b. psychological tests

c. experiments

d. laboratory observation

14. _____ are manipulated and assessed in scientific studies.

  a. Theories

  b. Variables

  c. Correlations

  d. Coefficients of correlation

15. Researchers manipulate the _____ variable to discover its effect on the _____ variable in an experiment.

  a. independent; dependent

  b. dependent; independent

  c. hypothesis; theory

  d. control group; experimental group

16. Random assignment is a procedure designed to ensure that individuals participating in an experiment will be

  a. more likely to be chosen for the experimental group.

  b. more likely to be chosen for the control group.

  c. just as likely to be chosen for the experimental group as the control group.

  d. more likely to be identified as unsuitable for either group.

17. In a double-blind study, _____ know which subjects are in the control group and which subjects are in the experimental group.

  a. only the researchers

  b. only the subjects

  c. neither the subjects nor the researchers

  d. both the subjects and the researchers

18. In the video program, the people tabulating the results of the cognitive interviews and the standard police interviews were not allowed to see the actual questions; this served as a kind of double-blind precaution to

  a. keep the experimenters from modifying the data.

  b. keep the transcribers from adding their own data.

  c. identify liars.

  d. prevent bias and ensure objectivity.

19. You'd be more likely to believe that research on the dating habits of college students could be applied to the real world

   a. even if the study's findings were unsubstantiated, but the research had been carried out by famous scientists.

   b. if the results of an experiment and of a survey confirmed one another.

   c. if you knew someone who had participated in such a study.

   d. if the conclusions of the study were based on extensive observations of laboratory animals.

20. If all of the subjects in a psychological research study were army enlisted personnel with 20 or more years of service, to which of the following matters would interpretation of the results be LEAST likely to apply?

   a. attitudes toward authority

   b. interest in physical fitness

   c. planning for retirement

   d. developing new technical skills to improve chances for promotion

21. Significance based on statistical evidence within a single study, even though it is scientifically obtained, compiled, and analyzed, _____ imply real-world importance.

   a. can never

   b. will always

   c. doesn't always

   d. may, if the statistical sample is large enough,

22. The APA (American Psychological Association) code of ethics calls on psychologists to respect the _____ and _____ of their subjects.

   a. privacy; desires

   b. dignity; welfare

   c. religious beliefs; political convictions

   d. friends; relatives

23. Ethical guidelines for psychological experiments call for human subjects to decide voluntarily to participate in a study and to know enough about it to make an intelligent decision, a doctrine known as

    a. voluntary self-deception.

    b. controlled consent.

    c. informed deception.

    d. informed consent.

24. Defenders of _____ research refuse to acknowledge that confinement in laboratories can be psychologically and physically harmful for some species.

    a. structuralist

    b. fundamentalist

    c. animal

    d. anti-intellectualistic

Study Activities

These activities challenge you to use your critical thinking and demonstrate how what you are learning can be applied to you and your own life. Try those activities that interest you most and/or those your instructor assigns.

1. Have you ever made a phone call or sent a letter or telegram to an elected representative to demand action on a particular issue? If so, have you later learned from the news that a certain number of constituents had registered their opinions in the same way and that such and such a percentage took the position you did? If you were in the majority, you probably felt pleased and justified in having taken the trouble to call or write. If yours was a minority position, you may have grumbled that most of the people sharing your viewpoint had probably failed to express their opinion; you and they were part of the "silent" majority.

    Similar informal polls on politics, sports, and various aspects of popular culture are growing in popularity; these include call-in surveys conducted by television or radio programs (often using "900" numbers that automatically count the calls, and for which there is a charge), which provide almost immediate totals and tabulations of the many calls received.

    Without thinking about whether or not such samplings of opinion were scientific, your instincts must have told you that the numbers reported were unlikely to reflect the views of the entire population. As a study activity, begin keeping a record of all the polls and surveys you encounter. Identify each poll and indicate if it appears to be scientifically designed and conducted.

    If a poll or survey seems unscientific, say why. Has the suspect survey failed to use a representative sample of the population it claims to study? Does it suffer from volunteer bias? Does it allow individuals to register their opinion more than once? Does its method favor people with more money (by having participants pay to be in the poll) or education (by having questions requiring knowledge beyond that of average people)? Does it make it particularly easy for participants safely to provide erroneous information? Look for these and any other signs that a poll or survey is unscientific, unreliable, untrustworthy, and unworthy of your involvement, attention, or concern.

2. Ethical questions are largely a matter of opinion; that is, the right answer for one person may be entirely wrong for someone else. Some difficult ethical issues face many scientists doing psychological research. Some people assert that it is wrong to use animals in research, to manipulate their behavior, attach

measurement devices to them, perform surgery to determine their reactions, and even kill them and examine their remains to discover how some experiment affected them. The opposing opinion states that progress toward the treatment and cure of most diseases depends on animal research, that people with cancer, diabetes, AIDS, and many other serious ailments would have no hope at all if researchers could not use animals to test their theories, surgical procedures, and medications.

Similarly, there is considerable disagreement about the use of deception in psychological research. There have been experiments in which some or all of the subjects did not know what the true purpose of the study was, or in which they did not know their behavior was being manipulated and studied. In some research, the impressive paraphernalia of scientific research and the authority of science and the scientist have encouraged experimental subjects to behave in ways that they would consider unacceptable, for themselves or others, outside the experimental setting.

Such research may produce some illuminating findings, but the ethical issues remain unresolved. Researchers must always consider when, if ever, it is right to tell lies as a means to obtaining the truth.

No study assignment in a psychology survey course is going to settle such daunting ethical questions. However, you can get involved in the issue; you can contribute to identifying and solving the problem. Your first task is vigilance. Pay attention to what researchers are doing in the name of science, truth, health, the future, the nation, the human race, and so on. Look for newspaper and magazine articles and radio and television coverage of stories concerning research and research methods (in all sciences). Be more concerned with media coverage of the research itself than with pieces on the controversy over an experiment or the way it was done. You want to collect data, facts, information—not more opinions about that information.

As you gather your information, analyze it in the light of what you've been learning in this course. As fairly and objectively as possible, try to decide where there are genuine ethical issues worthy of attention and debate. And, of course, before you allow yourself to be part of any research project, be sure you know what you're getting into. For example, the famous Milgram experiment on obedience to authority (which is covered in Lesson 24 of this telecourse) not only revealed that most subjects were willing to give the "learners" higher and higher shocks, but that only a very few subjects refused to give even the first, mildest, shock. In studying right and wrong behavior by researchers, it may well be that the moral imperative of not doing *any* harm is as worthy of consideration as the question of how much harm might be done to achieve a measure of good.

Lesson 3

The Biology of Behavior

Assignments

For the most systematic coverage of this lesson, we suggest that you complete the assignments in the sequence listed below.

Before viewing the video program:

- Read the "Learning Objectives" and "Overview" for this lesson. Use the Learning Objectives to guide your reading, viewing, and thinking.

- Read the "Viewing Notes" for this lesson.

- Read Chapter 4, "Neurons, Hormones, and the Brain," pages 99–112, 133–134, in the Wade and Tavris text. First, familiarize yourself with its contents by reading the Chapter Outline. As you read, note terms and concepts set in bold or italic type, especially those defined in the margins.

View the video program, "The Biology of Behavior"

After viewing the video program:

- Briefly note your answers to the questions at the end of the "Viewing Notes."

- Review all reading assignments for this lesson, including the Summary at the end of Chapter 4 in the textbook.

- Complete the "Review Exercises" to strengthen your understanding of this lesson's central concepts and terminology. Pay special attention to the "Vocabulary Check" exercise and the additional terms and concepts that follow—page references indicate where in the text assignment each term is defined. [Remember: there is a complete Glossary at the end of the text.]

- Take the "Self-Test" to measure the degree to which you are achieving this lesson's learning objectives. Check your answers against the "Answer Key" and review when necessary.

- Follow the suggestions in the "Study Activities" section at the end of this lesson and complete any other activities and projects assigned by your instructor.

Learning Objectives

When you have completed all assignments in this lesson, you should be able to:

1. Identify the basic components that make up the central nervous system and the peripheral nervous system.

2. Identify the two divisions of the autonomic nervous system and explain the function of each.

3. List and describe the major parts and functions of a neuron, and describe the process through which neurons communicate in the nervous system.

4. Identify several neurotransmitters and discuss their known or suspected effects.

5. Explain the basic function of hormones produced by the endocrine glands.

Overview

This lesson deals with the physical foundations of human behavior, with the biochemical processes underlying how and why we think, feel, act, and react as we do. It introduces the basic components of the nervous system and the many subdivisions of that system: the **central nervous system**, comprising the brain and spinal cord; the **peripheral nervous system**, composed of **motor nerves** and **sensory nerves** and divided into the **somatic nervous system**; and the **autonomic nervous system**. The **parasympathetic** and **sympathetic** divisions of the autonomic system, which play a crucial role in dealing with stress and threat, are described in detail.

The basic building blocks of the nervous system, **neurons** (or nerve cells), are described in great detail. Their constituent parts—the **axon, dendrites,** and **cell body**—are identified and their functions explained. The role of the **myelin sheath** and **action potential** in speeding up conduction of neural impulses is discussed. This lesson provides information on **neurotransmission**, the process by which electrochemical messages are transmitted throughout the nervous system, from neuron to neuron. You will learn how messages are carried by **neurotransmitters** across the **synaptic cleft**, the minuscule gap between the axon of one neuron and a dendrite or the cell body of another.

Both the textbook and the video program demonstrate the important role that neurotransmitters play in generating and controlling human behavior. They show how imbalances in neurotransmitters can contribute to many ailments, including Parkinson's disease, Alzheimer's disease, bipolar disorder (characterized by alternating episodes of depression and mania), schizophrenia, and childhood autism.

This lesson also explains that **hormones** as well as neurotransmitters affect how we act and feel. The nature and functions of the three principal sex hormones—**estrogens, androgens**, and **progesterone**—are described. Other hormones, such as melatonin and the adrenal hormones, are also discussed. Hormones and neurotransmitters are shown to interact as parts of the complex **neuroendocrine system** of chemical messengers.

Viewing Notes

The video program "The Biology of Behavior" describes the human nervous system as a "vast internal communications network which connects every part of our body to every other part." The program explains why that network evolved to its present state of intricacy and capability, a mechanism made up of billions of parts working together to keep us alive and aware. The program introduces the brain, other basic components of the nervous system, and the central process of communication: neurotransmission. It shows how the scientific understanding of the nervous system has depended on the study of unfortunate individuals whose nervous systems have been damaged or diseased. The noted scholars who appear in the program discuss the extent to which ongoing research into human physiology and biochemistry is revealing how the nervous system generates and regulates behavior.

As you watch the video program, consider the following questions:

1. What do we learn about the nature of the human nervous system from the behavior and responses of police officers experiencing stress in dangerous situations?

2. According to Arnold Scheibel, how do the components and processes of the nervous system produce behavior that keeps us out of trouble and gets us what we want?

3. Why does Scheibel believe that "threat is the impetus for maximal efficiency in the nervous system"?

4. How does Charles Woody describe neurotransmission?

5. What does Chris Gallen say about the role of neurotransmission in his patient Carl Armstrong's Parkinson's disease?

6. How is Floyd Bloom using computer imaging to understand neurons and neurotransmitters?

7. What does Bloom say about the relationship between neurotransmitters and hormones?

8. Why does Scheibel assert: "We essentially are our neurotransmitters"?

Review Exercises

Vocabulary Check

Match the following key terms and concepts with the appropriate definitions from the list below.

1. ____ androgens (p. 111)

2. ____ autonomic nervous system (p. 101; video)

3. ____ axon (p. 105; video)

4. ____ dendrites (p. 105; video)

5. ____ endorphins (p. 110)

6. ____ hormones (p. 111; video)

7. ____ motor nerves (p. 101)

8. ____ neuron (p. 103; video)

9. ____ neurotransmitter (p. 107; video)

10. ____ peripheral nervous system (p. 101)

11. ____ sensory nerves (p. 101)

12. ____ spinal reflex (p. 100)

13. ____ sympathetic nervous system (p. 102)

14. ____ synapse (p. 107)

a. the portion of the nervous system outside the brain and spinal cord

b. automatic response to a stimulus

c. nerves in the peripheral nervous system that carry messages toward the central nervous system

d. nerves in the peripheral nervous system that carry messages from the central nervous system to muscles, glands, and internal organs

e. subdivision of the peripheral nervous system that regulates the internal organs and glands

f. subdivision of the autonomic nervous system that mobilizes bodily resources and increases the output of energy during emotion and stress (the so-called fight-or-flight response)

g. cell that conducts electrochemical messages; basic unit of the nervous system; also called a nerve cell

h. branches on a neuron that receive information from other nerve cells and transmit it toward the cell body

i. that part of a neuron which conducts impulses away from the cell body and transmits them to other nerve cells

j. the site where transmission of a nerve impulse from one nerve cell to another occurs

k. a chemical substance that is released by a transmitting neuron at the synapse and alters the activity of a receiving neuron

l. human neurotransmitters similar in structure and action to opiates such as heroin and morphine

m. chemical substances secreted by organs called glands and that affect the functioning of other organs

n. masculinizing hormones

Other Key Terms and Concepts

action potential (p. 107; video)

adrenal hormones (p. 111)

biofeedback (p. 101)

cell body (p. 105; video)

central nervous system (p. 100; video)

endocrine glands (p. 111; video)

estrogens (p. 111)

excitation and inhibition in the nervous system (p. 107; video)

glial cells (p. 103)

melatonin (p. 111)

myelin sheath (p. 105)

nerves (p. 105)

neuromodulators (p. 110)

parasympathetic nervous system (p. 102)

progesterone (p. 111)

sex hormones (p. 111)

somatic nervous system (p. 101; video)

spinal cord (p. 100)

synaptic vesicles (p. 107)

Completion

Fill each blank with the most appropriate term from the list of answers below.

15. The brain and spinal cord constitute the _____ nervous system.

16. The _____ nervous system works without a person's conscious control.

17. The skeletal nervous system is another name for the _____ nervous system.

18. _____ is a technique for controlling a bodily function through use of an instrument that monitors that function and signals changes in it.

19. The _____ division of the autonomic nervous system mobilizes the body in the face of emotion and stress, whereas the _____ division operates when the body is in more relaxed states.

20. _____ cells hold _____ in place and provide them with nutrients.

21. The _____ are branches of the neuron that receive information and transmit it toward the _____ body.

22. The axons of many neurons have a fatty insulation called the _____.

23. Dopamine, serotonin, and acetylcholine are all _____.

24. _____, chambers at the tip of an axon, contain neurotransmitter molecules.

25. The neurotransmitters known as endogenous opioid peptides, or more popularly as _____, have painkilling and pleasure-promoting effects similar to those of such drugs as _____ and morphine.

26. Hormones are chemical substances that originate primarily in the _____, which deposit them in the _____ to be carried to organs and cells throughout the body.

27. _____, which is secreted by the pineal body, a small gland deep within the brain, appears to regulate certain biological rhythms.

28. The physical changes in males at puberty are produced by sex hormones called _____ and the changes in females at puberty are produced by sex hormones called _____.

androgens	endocrine glands	neurons
autonomic	endorphins	neurotransmitters
biofeedback	estrogens	parasympathetic
bloodstream	glial	somatic
cell	heroin	sympathetic
central	melatonin	synaptic vesicles
dendrites	myelin sheath	

True-False

Read the following statements carefully and mark each true (T) or false (F).

29. ___ Neuropsychology is principally devoted to the study of how endocrine glands and hormones influence behavior.

30. ___ The central nervous system processes, interprets, and stores incoming sensory information and sends out orders to muscles, glands, and body organs.

31. ___ Sensory nerves receive signals indicating the need for some action and instruct the appropriate muscles, glands, or internal organs to function.

32. ___ The peripheral nervous system comprises two subdivisions: the somatic nervous system and the autonomic nervous system.

33. ___ After you have carefully analyzed an uncertain situation, you may decide to activate your sympathetic nervous system, which will mobilize the body's resources to deal with the stress and emotion of a threat or emergency.

34. ___ All neurons are basically the same size and shape.

35. ___ The dendrites of a neuron receive messages from other nerve cells, and the axon transmits messages to other cells.

36. ___ The strength with which individual neurons fire can vary enormously.

37. ___ Some endorphins function as neurotransmitters, but most act primarily as neuromodulators, which increase or decrease the action of specific neurotransmitters.

38. ___ Hormones and neurotransmitters function independently of one another.

39. ___ There are three types of human sex hormones, and all three occur in both males and females.

Short-Answer Questions

As a final review exercise, write brief answers to demonstrate that you are achieving the learning objectives of this lesson.

1. Identify the basic components that make up the central nervous system and the peripheral nervous system.

2. Identify the two divisions of the autonomic nervous system and explain the function of each.

3. List and describe the major parts and functions of a neuron, and describe the process through which neurons communicate in the nervous system.

4. Identify several neurotransmitters and discuss their known or suspected effects.

5. Explain the basic function of hormones produced by the endocrine glands.

Self-Test

1. The central nervous system is made up of
    a.   axons and dendrites.
    b.   the brain and the spinal cord.
    c.   the autonomic and somatic nervous systems.
    d.   the sympathetic and parasympathetic nervous systems.

2. The spinal cord is an extension of the
    a.   brain.
    b.   neuroendocrine system.
    c.   skeletal system.
    d.   spinal column.

3. In the peripheral nervous system, messages are carried to and from the central nervous system by
    a.   neurotransmitters.
    b.   hormones.
    c.   biofeedback.
    d.   sensory nerves and motor nerves, respectively.

4. The peripheral nervous system is made up of
    a.   axons and dendrites.
    b.   the brain and the spinal cord.
    c.   the autonomic and somatic nervous systems.
    d.   the sympathetic and parasympathetic nervous systems.

5. The autonomic nervous system is made up of
    a.   axons and dendrites.
    b.   the brain and the spinal cord.
    c.   sensory nerves only.
    d.   the sympathetic and parasympathetic nervous systems.

6. The two parts of the autonomic nervous system
   a. function under the conscious direction of the brain.
   b. may cease to function under the pressure of stress and emotion.
   c. work together, but in opposing ways, to adjust the body to changing circumstances.
   d. are independent systems perpetually struggling to control a person's moods and behavior.

7. The subdivision of the autonomic nervous system that is like the accelerator of a car, enabling your body to go faster and put out more energy, is the
   a. sympathetic division.
   b. parasympathetic division.
   c. adrenal gland division.
   d. motor nerve division.

8. The subdivision of the autonomic nervous system that is like the brake of a car, tending to slow your body down and conserve energy, is the
   a. sympathetic division.
   b. parasympathetic division.
   c. adrenal gland division.
   d. motor nerve division.

9. The major parts of a neuron include each of the following **EXCEPT** the
   a. dendrites.
   b. axon.
   c. synaptic cleft.
   d. glial cells.

10. The cell body of a neuron
    a. conducts impulses away from the cell body and transmits them to other neurons.
    b. receives information from other neurons and transmits it toward the cell body.
    c. keeps the neuron alive and determines whether or not it fires.
    d. manufactures and stores neurotransmitters.

11. The function of dendrites is to
    a. conduct impulses away from the cell body and transmit them to other neurons.
    b. receive information from other neurons and transmit it toward the cell body.
    c. keep the neuron alive and determine whether or not it will fire.
    d. manufacture and store neurotransmitters.

12. The function of the axon is to
    a. conduct impulses away from the cell body and transmit them to other neurons or to muscle or gland cells.
    b. receive information from other neurons and transmit it toward the cell body.
    c. keep the neuron alive and determine whether or not it will fire.
    d. manufacture and store neurotransmitters.

13. Bundles of fibers (axons and sometimes dendrites) in the peripheral nervous system are called
    a. glial cells.
    b. tracts.
    c. nodes.
    d. nerves.

14. Neurotransmission, the method neurons use to communicate in the nervous system, involves
    a. conscious control requiring considerable effort and learning.
    b. an electrochemical process in which chemical substances travel from the axon of one neuron across a synapse to a dendrite or cell body of another nerve cell.
    c. stimulation of the endocrine glands to produce hormones that carry messages and instructions throughout the body.
    d. reflexes acquired over years of stimulation and response.

15. Low levels of _____ have been associated with severe depression.
    a. serotonin and norepinephrine
    b. endorphins and dopamine
    c. serotonin and acetylcholine
    d. epinephrine and norepinephrine

16. A deficiency in the neurotransmitter _____ has been implicated in Alzheimer's disease.
    a. dopamine
    b. serotonin
    c. acetylcholine
    d. GABA

In the blank next to each of the following definitions, write the letter of the most appropriate term or concept from the list that follows.

17. ____ the minuscule space across which neurotransmitters carry messages

18. ____ the substance that some people suffering from Parkinson's disease have undergone experimental surgery to obtain by means of grafts of brain and adrenal gland tissue that produces it

19. ____ the nervous system's opiatelike neuromodulators, which relieve pain and produce pleasure

20. ____ the major inhibitory neurotransmitter in the brain

    a. GABA   c. dopamine
    b. endorphins   d. synaptic cleft (gap)

21. The basic function of hormones is to
    a. regulate metabolism.
    b. affect how body organs function.
    c. promote growth and direct sexual development.
    d. counteract the influence of neurotransmitters.

22. Hormones carry their messages throughout the body by means of
   a. the bloodstream.
   b. neurotransmission.
   c. the reflex arc.
   d. synaptic vesicles.

23. The parts of the nervous and endocrine systems that interact are often referred to as the
   a. synaptic vesicles.
   b. sympathetic nervous system.
   c. parasympathetic nervous system.
   d. neuroendocrine system.

24. Two adrenal hormones that also appear to function as neurotransmitters in the brain are
   a. dopamine and serotonin.
   b. progesterone and testosterone.
   c. epinephrine and norepinephrine.
   d. insulin and toblerone.

25. The three main types of sex hormones are
   a. endorphins, enkephalins, and dynorphins.
   b. androgens, estrogens, and progesterone.
   c. cortisol, epinephrine, and norepinephrine.
   d. insulin, thyroxin, and melatonin.

Study Activities

These activities challenge you to use your critical thinking and demonstrate how what you are learning can be applied to you and your own life. Try those activities that interest you most and/or those your instructor assigns.

1. Review the boxed passage "Taking Psychology with You—Food for Thought: Diet and Neurotransmitters" on pages 133–134 of the Wade and Tavris textbook. Consider what it reveals about the possible links between diet and behavior. Ask yourself if what it describes applies to you or to any of your friends or family; that is, do you or people you know try to eat foods that purportedly influence health, mood, or performance?

   As a study activity, keep a written record over one or two weeks of everything you eat. Pay particular attention to items you've made part of your diet largely or entirely because of something you've read, seen on television, or been told. For instance, indicate if you attempt to limit your intake of sodium (salt), sugar, fats and cholesterol, or red meat. Record your efforts to increase your consumption of such things as oat bran, vegetables, and fish. Honestly examine your eating habits to identify the degree to which your diet contains nutrients, vitamin and mineral supplements, fad foods, and health foods you believe—or want to believe—can make you healthier, stronger, calmer, better able to sleep, more energetic, and so on.

   Repeat this activity at the end of the semester to see if your diet is fairly stable or if new fads and food passions have altered your eating habits.

2. The video program "The Biology of Behavior" shows police trainees learning to deal with various threats and emergencies. They are placed in stressful situations, facing unknown individuals. In some cases, the officers may have to use their weapons against armed felons; in others, they must refrain from accidentally harming innocent bystanders in the excitement of the moment. The text explains that the sympathetic division of the human nervous system responds to emotion and threat by mobilizing the body's resources. It also points out that the parasympathetic nervous system keeps that mobilization from getting out of control. It serves as a brake, working with the sympathetic division to allow individuals to cope with stressful encounters and still maintain the control—as in the case of police officers—to act appropriately but refrain from hurting themselves or the citizens they are supposed to protect.

From your own experience, recall occasions when you were subjected to sufficient emotional excitement or physical threat to activate the kind of stress reaction described in the text and the video lesson. Perhaps you were in an auto accident, or had a very close call. Maybe you felt extremely agitated at the prospect of a job interview or had some equally exciting experience that involved facing a threat or coping with expectations. Remember how it felt, both while it was happening and later, when you were calming down. Write down as much as you can remember. Record whether and when your palms and your mouth were wet or dry; describe your heart rate, how your stomach felt, and any changes in your vision or in your sense of well-being.

The idea is to increase your awareness of your body's system for dealing with stress. That system has been central to the survival of human beings, both as individuals and as a species. By increasing your personal knowledge of the subject, you will not only improve your understanding of an important aspect of psychology (Lesson 19 is devoted entirely to this subject) but also should improve your day-to-day coping skills.

The Brain-Mind Connection

Assignments

For the most systematic coverage of this lesson, we suggest that you complete the assignments in the sequence listed below.

Before viewing the video program:

- Read the "Learning Objectives" and "Overview" for this lesson. Use the Learning Objectives to guide your reading, viewing, and thinking.

- Read the "Viewing Notes" for this lesson.

- Read Chapter 4, "Neurons, Hormones, and the Brain," pages 113–133, in the Wade and Tavris text. First, familiarize yourself with its contents by reading the Chapter Outline. As you read, note terms and concepts set in bold or italic type, especially those defined in the margins.

View the video program, "The Brain-Mind Connection"

After viewing the video program:

- Briefly note your answers to the questions at the end of the "Viewing Notes."

- Review all reading assignments for this lesson, including the Summary at the end of Chapter 4 in the textbook.

- Complete the "Review Exercises" to strengthen your understanding of this lesson's central concepts and terminology. Pay special attention to the "Vocabulary Check" exercise and the additional terms and concepts that follow—page references indicate where in the text assignment each term is defined. [Remember: there is a complete Glossary at the end of the text.]

- Take the "Self-Test" to measure the degree to which you are achieving this lesson's learning objectives. Check your answers against the "Answer Key" and review when necessary.

- Follow the suggestions in the "Study Activities" section at the end of this lesson and complete any other activities and projects assigned by your instructor.

Learning Objectives

When you have completed all assignments in this lesson, you should be able to:

1. Describe how the following devices are used by researchers to study living brains: EEG (electroencephalogram), PET scan (positron-emission tomography), and MRI (magnetic resonance imaging).

2. Identify and describe the major structures and functions of the hindbrain, midbrain, and forebrain.

3. Describe the key functions of the limbic system.

4. Discuss the importance of the cerebral cortex; describe key functions of the occipital, parietal, temporal, and frontal lobes.

5. Describe the effect of split-brain operations on patients' perception and language.

6. Explain the concept of localization of function as well as those theories that suggest the brain be viewed as an integrated whole.

7. Discuss the controversies over whether or not there are physical differences between the brains of human females and human males and over whether these and other differences between brains are present at birth or may result from environmental or social influences.

Overview

The human brain is the subject of this lesson. This extraordinary organ is examined in detail to explain what makes it more powerful than the brains of any other animals. The various structures of the brain are described and their functions explained.

The major sections of the brain and their principal structures are discussed. The **brain stem** and **hindbrain**—comprising the **medulla**, the **pons**, the **reticular activating system** (**RAS**), and the **cerebellum**—are identified as vital to keeping the body alive and crucial to fundamental mental functions. The forebrain, the largest portion of the brain, is described in detail, showing how the actions of its constituent elements make each of us human and uniquely ourselves. The lesson explains the roles of the **thalamus**, **hypothalamus**, and **pituitary gland** in regulating critical bodily functions and the involvement of the **limbic system** in basic emotional reactions and motivated behavior.

Special attention is given to the cerebral cortex, that portion of the brain responsible for thought, creativity, speech, and all the other "higher" mental functions. The key functions of the four lobes of the cortex—the **occipital**, **parietal**, **temporal**, and **frontal**—are identified. The fascinating subject of the apparent differences between the functions and capabilities of the right and left hemispheres of the brain is examined in the text and, quite movingly and informatively, in the video program. There is coverage of both the so-called **split-brain operations** and **hemispherectomies**. The issues of **hemispheric dominance** and **localization of function** are explored. There is discussion of conflicting theories that contend specific functions are centered in certain areas of the brain or that hold various functions are distributed over many areas or throughout the whole brain.

The text and video program confront the controversy over the origin and extent of differences between individuals' brains—especially the reported differences between the brains of men and of women. The opposing viewpoints are presented, giving you the opportunity to decide for yourself which perspective is more convincing: that differences arise from genetic factors present at birth or that social and environmental influences shape the physical brain and intellectual functioning. You are prompted to consider what, if anything, differences have to do with an individual's behavior.

The lesson also describes some of the remarkable devices being used to study the living human brain, both for medical diagnosis and to advance knowledge about the nature and workings of the brain. There are passages on the **electroencephalogram** (**EEG**), the **PET scan** (**positron-emission tomography**), and **magnetic resonance imaging** (**MRI**).

Viewing Notes

The "Brain-Mind Connection" video program explores the ways in which the physical attributes of the brain influence and are influenced by thought, behavior, culture, and the environment. It provides vivid examples of why the human brain has been called "the most complicated biological organ on the face of the earth." That is the way neurobiologist Arnold Scheibel characterizes the brain when he appears in this program—holding a real brain in his hands and explaining the basic structures and functions of the miraculous three-pound organ on which every human thought and action depends. This video lesson raises intriguing questions about the nature and limits of human mental capacity, about where particular mental functions are located in the brain, and about whether or not apparent physical differences between the brains of human males and those of females are the result of genetic or social and environmental forces.

As you watch the video program, consider the following questions:

1. What do the experiences of Guy Gabelich (the little boy who underwent a hemispherectomy) suggest about the human brain's plasticity: its ability to adapt?

2. What does Dr. Harry Chugani say about the relationship between Guy's age at the time of the operation and his ability to recover from having half his cerebral cortex removed?

3. Is plasticity characteristic only of young brains that have undergone major trauma, or do normal brains also change in response to the environment both during development and throughout the life span?

4. As he is describing the various areas and structures of the brain, what does Arnold Scheibel say about specialization or localization of function?

5. What has the research of Dahlia Zaidel, Eran Zaidel, and Jeffrey Clarke revealed about the specialization (or generalization) of functions between the right and left cerebral hemispheres and about how the hemispheres communicate with each other?

6. What are some of Marian Diamond's research findings on the differences between the brains of female rats and those of male rats?

7. Why does Marsha Linn assert that environmental and social influences are more likely than genetic factors to be responsible for reported differences in intellectual ability between men and women?

8. How may Diamond's studies of the effects of an enriched environment on the physical growth of rats' brains relate to human cognitive development in childhood and later life?

Review Exercises

Vocabulary Check

Match the following key terms and concepts with the appropriate definitions from the list below.

1. __D__ brain stem (p. 117)

2. ____ cerebral cortex (p. 120)

3. ____ corpus callosum (p. 120)

4. __A__ electroencephalogram (EEG) (p. 113)

5. ____ hemispheric dominance or specialization (pp. 127–128; video)

6. ____ hypothalamus (p. 117)

7. ____ limbic system (p. 118)

8. ____ localization of function (p. 116; video)

9. ____ magnetic resonance imaging (MRI) (p. 114; video)

10. ____ occipital lobes (p. 120)

11. ____ pituitary gland (p. 118)

12. ____ positron-emission tomography (PET scan) (p. 114; video)

13. ____ reticular activating system (RAS) (p. 117)

14. ____ split-brain surgery (pp. 124–125)

15. ____ temporal lobes (p. 120)

a. a recording of neural activity detected by electrodes

b. a method for analyzing biochemical activity in the brain, using injections of a glucose-like substance containing a radioactive element

c. a method for studying body and brain tissue, using magnetic fields and special radio receivers

d. the part of the brain, at the top of the spinal cord, responsible for automatic functions such as heartbeat and respiration

e. dense network of neurons in the core of the brain stem; arouses higher centers of the brain and screens incoming information

f. brain structure involved in emotions and drives vital to survival, such as fear, hunger, thirst, and reproduction; controls the autonomic nervous system

g. the body's "master gland"

h. group of brain areas involved in emotional reactions and motivated behavior

i. the part of the brain responsible for such higher functions as thought and creativity

j. the area of the cortex, in the back of the brain, that processes visual signals

k. areas of the cortex, on the sides of the brain, that process auditory signals and are involved in memory, perception, emotion, and language comprehension

l. the large band of nerve fibers that connects the two cerebral hemispheres and that is severed in a split-brain operation

m. the notion that one cerebral hemisphere, usually the left one in most right-handed people, predominates in processing language and handling most logical, sequential tasks

n. different brain parts perform different (though overlapping) tasks

o. a medical procedure in which the corpus callosum is cut, severing the connection between the two cerebral hemispheres

Other Key Terms and Concepts

amygdala (p. 119)

association cortex (p. 121)

auditory cortex (p. 120)

Broca's area (p. 121)

cerebellum (p. 117)

cerebral hemispheres
    (p. 120; video)

cerebrum (p. 120)

electrodes (p. 114)

frontal lobes (p. 120)

hemispherectomy (video)

hippocampus (p. 119)

"his" and "hers" brains
    (pp. 130–132; video)

lateralization (p. 120; video)

medulla (p. 117)

motor cortex (p. 121)

parietal lobes (p. 120)

plasticity (p. 107; video)

pons (p. 117)

prefrontal cortex (p. 121)

somatosensory cortex
    (p. 120)

thalamus (p. 117)

visual cortex (p. 120)

Wernicke's area (p. 120)

Completion

Fill each blank with the most appropriate term from the list of answers below.

16. _____ are devices used to apply electrical current to tissue or to detect neural activity.

17. The imaging technique that records biochemical changes in the brain is called _____, and the technique that produces vibrations in the nuclei of the atoms making up body organs is _____.

18. The major subdivisions of the hindbrain are the brain stem—comprising the _____ and the _____—the _____ system (RAS), and the _____.

19. Behaviors that are largely reflexive or automatic are likely to be controlled by areas in the _____ and _____, whereas control of more complex behavior is usually centered in the _____.

20. The _____ is the brain's "thinking cap": the center of higher mental processes such as thought, planning, and creativity.

21. Personality has long been associated with the _____ lobes of the cortex.

22. In almost all right-handed people, the _____ hemisphere is usually "dominant" over the _____ hemisphere, and nearly all right-handers and most left-handers process _____ in the left hemisphere.

23. The guiding principle of modern brain theories is _____, which emphasizes the specialization of areas and structures of the brain; minority _____ views hold that information is distributed throughout the brain.

24. Research shows physical differences between the brains of _____, but conclusions based on these findings remain highly controversial.

25. Physical differences between human brains and in intellectual abilities may be as attributable to _____ and _____ influences as to genetic factors.

cerebellum

cerebral cortex

electrodes

environmental

forebrain

frontal

hindbrain

holistic

human males and
females

language

left

localization of
function

magnetic resonance
imaging (MRI)

medulla

midbrain

pons

positron-emission
tomography
(PET scan)

reticular activating

right

social

True-False

Read the following statements carefully and mark each true (T) or false (F).

26. ___ An electroencephalogram (EEG) describes the structure and function of the brain more precisely than any other means.

27. ___ The cerebrum is the largest brain structure and handles most sensory, motor, and cognitive processes.

28. ___ The pituitary gland, like the appendix, no longer plays any apparent purpose in the working of the human body.

29. ___ The limbic system contains the so-called pleasure areas of the brain.

30. ___ Most areas of the cerebral cortex are "silent"; that is, nothing happens after they are electrically stimulated.

31. ___ Few "split-brain" patients ever regain their ability to walk, talk, or lead otherwise normal lives.

32. ___ All brain researchers agree that the left hemisphere of the brain is dominant and more important than the right hemisphere.

33. ___ Many of the differences observed between the anatomy of the brains of male rats and those of females closely parallel differences between the brains of male and female humans.

34. ___ There is growing evidence that the individuality of brain networks exceeds that of fingerprints or facial features.

35. ___ An individual's experiences may play a role in shaping the physical organization of his or her brain.

Short-Answer Questions

As a final review exercise, write brief answers to demonstrate that you are achieving the learning objectives of this lesson.

1. Describe how the following devices are used by researchers to study living brains: EEG (electroencephalogram), PET scan (positron-emission tomography), and MRI (magnetic resonance imaging).

2. Identify and describe the major structures and functions of the hindbrain, midbrain, and forebrain.

3. Describe the key functions of the limbic system.

4. Discuss the importance of the cerebral cortex; describe key functions of the occipital, parietal, temporal, and frontal lobes.

5. Describe the effect of split-brain operations on patients' perception and language.

6. Explain the concept of localization of function as well as those theories that suggest the brain be viewed as an integrated whole.

7. Discuss the controversies over whether or not there are physical differences between the brains of human females and human males and over whether these and other differences between brains are present at birth or may result from environmental or social influences.

Self-Test

1. Researchers wishing to study the brain's electrical wave patterns would want to use

   a. an electroencephalogram.

   b. a PET scan (positron-emission tomography).

   c. magnetic resonance imaging (MRI).

   d. X rays.

2. Positron-emission tomography (PET scan) provides

   a. recordings of electrical brain waves.

   b. images of living body and brain tissue.

   c. a record of the brain's biochemical activity.

   d. pictures of the inside of the skull and other bony structures surrounding the brain.

3. Magnetic resonance imaging (MRI) makes it easier to diagnose disease and study brain activity by

   a. locating metallic objects or substances in the brain.

   b. analyzing brain activity patterns, or evoked potentials.

   c. recording the brain's biochemical activity.

   d. revealing specific brain structures in detail.

4. This dense network of neurons extends from the core of the brain stem, filters out irrelevant incoming signals, and passes important information along to the higher centers of the brain.

   a. medulla

   b. pons

   c. reticular activating system (RAS)

   d. cerebellum

5. The _____, which is situated at the back of the hindbrain, plays a role in your sense of balance, helps coordinate muscle use and movement, and—according to some researchers—plays a role in higher cognitive functions such as analyzing sensory information and performing mental tasks such as solving puzzles or generating words.

   a. medulla

   b. pons

   c. reticular activating system (RAS)

   d. cerebellum

6. Two parts of the forebrain connected by a short stalk are the

   a. hypothalamus and the pituitary gland.

   b. hippocampus and the thyroid gland.

   c. cerebrum and the cerebellum.

   d. olfactory bulb and the thalamus.

7. The limbic system is a group of brain areas primarily

   a. movement and balance.

   b. higher cognitive processes.

   c. emotional reactions and motivated behavior.

   d. language comprehension.

8. Which structure in the limbic system may signal the brain's arousal center, the reticular activating system (RAS), to calm down about something that the RAS considered worthy of attention?

   a. hypothalamus

   b. hippocampus

   c. amygdala

   d. thalamus

9. Which structure in the limbic system is shaped like a sea horse and is called the "gateway to memory"?

    a. hypothalamus

    b. hippocampus

    c. amygdala

    d. thalamus

10. That layer of densely packed gray matter which contains almost three-quarters of all the cells in the human brain.

    a. occipital lobes

    b. association cortex

    c. cerebellum

    d. cerebral cortex

11. The _____ lobes contain the somatosensory cortex, which receives information about touch, pressure, pain, and temperature from all over the body.

    a. occipital

    b. parietal

    c. temporal

    d. frontal

12. The _____ lobes are involved in memory, perception, emotion, and language comprehension; they contain the auditory cortex.

    a. occipital

    b. parietal

    c. temporal

    d. frontal

13. If your frontal lobes were diseased or damaged, you would be most likely to experience an impairment in your ability to

    a. plan, think creatively, and show initiative.

    b. hear, remember, and express emotion.

    c. see.

    d analyze sensory experiences such as pain and temperature.

14. Split-brain operations were initially tried on humans as a last resort in coping with severe cases of

    a. schizophrenia.

    b. drug addiction.

    c. Parkinson's disease.

    d. epilepsy.

15. When the gaze of a split-brain patient is directed at a picture, half of which shows one person's face and the other half shows another face, each side of the patient's brain sees

    a. both faces, but can't describe what it sees.

    b. both faces, but must describe them either entirely through speech or entirely through pointing, gestures, or drawings.

    c. only one face and doesn't know what the other half of the brain sees.

    d. only one face, but also knows what the other half of the brain sees.

16. In split-brain patients, how does the dominant brain hemisphere (usually the left, which processes language and handles logical, sequential tasks) cope with the fact that some information is perceived only by the other hemisphere?

    a. It allows the other hemisphere to be "dominant" concerning such information.

    b. It makes up explanations based solely on its own perception.

    c. It finds new ways, including building new neural pathways, to communicate with the other hemisphere.

    d. It shows no awareness of or interest in the fact that the other hemisphere has separate perceptions.

17. Which of the following does **NOT** support the concept of localization of function?

    a. Specific centers of the brain are associated with specific functions.

    b. Some forms of knowledge may be dispersed throughout the entire brain.

    c. Specific nerve cells have specialized functions.

    d. Damage to even very small areas of the brain can have devastating effects.

In the blank next to each of the following definitions, write the letter of the most appropriate answer from the list that follows.

18. ___ term describing the concept that neural changes associated with individual thoughts, memories, and perceptions are confined to specific areas of the brain

19. ___ brain's capacity to adjust even after a major injury and/or operation and find new ways to function

    a. plasticity   c. localized

    b. holistic   d. distributed

20. Brain researchers such as Marian Diamond have discovered that

    a. no significant differences can be found between the brains of males and females—animal or human.

    b. the physical differences between male and female rat brains seem related to reproduction and sex hormones.

    c. enriched environments affect the brains of males only.

    d. environmental and social factors have no impact on brain development.

21. When it comes to explaining how brain differences between men and women are related to general intellectual ability,

    a. high-tech research methods have clarified how brain organization and chemistry affect human abilities.

    b. not many people are willing to theorize or speculate.

    c. most researchers are motivated solely by social and political purposes.

    d. no one has an entirely convincing theory.

22. The views of many popular writers on sex differences in the human brain are

    a. supported by considerable evidence and consequently are undeniable.

    b. little more than meaningless stereotypes.

    c. well established and generally accepted by the scientific community.

    d. motivated by the fact that women hold more of the same kinds of jobs as men hold.

23. Brain organization (the proportion of brain cells found in any particular part of the brain)

    a. is generally agreed to be genetically determined.

    b. depends mostly on environmental and cultural factors.

    c. is largely the same from person to person.

    d. varies considerably from person to person.

24. Theorists trying to create the most illuminating description of the nature and workings of the human brain would probably rely ón all but which one of the following?

    a. information on individuals' personal perception and experience

    b. traditional conceptions and widely held beliefs

    c. the physiological findings of brain scientists

    d. data on environmental and cultural influences

Study Activities

The following activity challenges you to use your critical thinking and demonstrate how what you are learning can be applied to you and your own life. Try this activity and/or others your instructor assigns.

Men and women are different in many ways. There are obvious physical differences, there are usually important differences in how any given society expects males and females to behave. The text chapter raises the intriguing issue of basic differences between the brains of human males and those of females. Using your own experience and reading for reference, consider the question of "his" and "hers" brains. Because experts still strongly disagree over whether such differences really exist and, if they exist, about whether they are due to genetic factors or cultural and environmental influences, you cannot be expected to make informed decisions about those aspects of the matter. But you can think about what you have done, observed, and thought.

Give examples of situations in which you've had the strong conviction that the ways in which members of the opposite sex think differ significantly from the ways individuals of your gender use their mind. From your own experience, can you honestly say that most men or women appear more "intellectual, creative, artistic, emotional, ingenious, strong-willed, and so on" than most members of the opposite sex? For instance, have you ever noticed that when both a man and a woman attempt to do the same thing or to solve the same problem they use different approaches or solutions? Have you seen men respond to a crisis or a challenge or a setback or a disappointment in markedly different ways from how women respond to identical stressful or demanding circumstances or events? Think about people you know best: your parents, brothers and sisters, close friends, your spouse, or anyone else you've been close to for long enough to observe the subtleties and particularities of their behavior and manner of thought. Don't forget to think about yourself and how you think and behave. Using specific examples, try to judge as coolly and impartially as you can whether or not you've detected evidence that men's brains and women's brains function in different ways.

Document instances of such things to produce your informal, personal survey of male-female differences. Be careful not to let the power of stereotypes confuse your efforts to gather convincing evidence. Pay special attention to instances of individuals behaving in ways that stereotypes ascribe almost exclusively to members of the other sex. Watch for men crying, women being aggressive, men being intuitive, women being analytical, and men being nurturing. Try to keep your survey going at least through the duration of this course. By doing so you will build a body of information to help you draw more trustworthy conclusions about the problem. The exercise will sharpen your skills as an observer of others and of your own attitudes and behavior.

Lesson 5

Body Rhythms and Mental States

Assignments

For the most systematic coverage of this lesson, we suggest that you complete the assignments in the sequence listed below.

Before viewing the video program:

- Read the "Learning Objectives" and "Overview" for this lesson. Use the Learning Objectives to guide your reading, viewing, and thinking.

- Read the "Viewing Notes" for this lesson.

- Read Chapter 5, "Body Rhythms and Mental States," in the Wade and Tavris text. First, familiarize yourself with its contents by reading the Chapter Outline. As you read, note terms and concepts set in bold or italic type, especially those defined in the margins.

View the video program, "Sleep and Dreaming"

After viewing the video program:

- Briefly note your answers to the questions at the end of the "Viewing Notes."

- Review all reading assignments for this lesson, including the Summary at the end of Chapter 5 in the textbook.

- Complete the "Review Exercises" to strengthen your understanding of this lesson's central concepts and terminology. Pay special attention to the "Vocabulary Check" exercise and the additional terms and concepts that follow—page references indicate where in the text assignment each term is defined. [Remember: there is a complete Glossary at the end of the text.]

- Take the "Self-Test" to measure the degree to which you are achieving this lesson's learning objectives. Check your answers against the "Answer Key" and review when necessary.

- Follow the suggestions in the "Study Activities" section at the end of this lesson and complete any other activities and projects assigned by your instructor.

Learning Objectives

When you have completed all assignments in this lesson, you should be able to:

1. Define and provide examples of biological rhythms, and explain why psychologists are interested in studying them.

2. Describe REM sleep and the four stages of non-REM sleep, and explain the pattern of the sleep cycle.

3. Discuss dreaming and the major explanations of why we dream: the psychoanalytic explanation, dreams as problem solving, dreams as information processing, and the activation-synthesis theory.

4. Discuss the common effects of psychoactive drugs and the results of abusing or being addicted to stimulant, depressant, opiate, and psychedelic drugs.

5. Explain how physical condition, past usage of a drug, mental set, and environmental setting can affect an individual's response to a drug.

6. Describe the general nature of hypnosis and provide examples of how hypnosis is used in medicine and psychology.

Overview

Everyone has intimate and extensive knowledge of the topics covered in this lesson. Everyone has experienced various **states of consciousness** and is familiar with many of the **biological rhythms** described. For example, the wake-sleep cycle is a **circadian rhythm** through which we all pass every day. Virtually all women have years of experience with at least one **infradian rhythm**, the menstrual cycle. This lesson describes these and other biological rhythms and explains why psychologists are interested in them.

The lesson pays particular attention to sleep and dreaming. The stages of sleep and what brain waves (such as **alpha** and **delta waves**) tell us about those stages are explained, and the special role and character of **REM** (**rapid eye movement**) sleep is explored. The text and video program discuss the major theories about what dreaming is and why we dream: the **psychoanalytic explanation**, **dreams as problem solving**, the **information-processing theory**, and **dreams as brain activity** (the **activation-synthesis theory**).

The common effects of **psychoactive drugs** and the results of abusing or being addicted to **stimulants**, **depressants**, **opiates**, and **psychedelics** are examined. The lesson also explains how a person's **physical condition**, **experience with a drug**, **mental set**, and the **environmental setting** can affect the way he or she responds to a drug.

The video program presents a number of researchers whose studies are helping to determine the nature and purposes of sleep and dreaming and to discover the causes and possible treatments for various sleep disorders.

The nature of **hypnosis** is discussed, with reference to recent studies that are allowing researchers supporting the major contending theories to agree on many issues. Examples are given of how hypnosis is used in research and to treat various ailments, help eliminate unwanted habits, improve performance, and build confidence. It is explained that medical professionals, as well as psychologists, have found hypnosis to be an intriguing process and a tool that can be used effectively for many medical and psychological purposes.

Viewing Notes

The video program for this lesson provides vivid examples of some of the biological rhythms and mental states explained in the text assignment. Experts discuss the medical and psychological aspects of sleep, identifying the most convincing theories of why we sleep and dream.

The program, "Sleep and Dreaming," deals not only with theories and experiments but also with practical matters of how sleep, dreams, and body rhythms influence our lives. It shows how and why an individual's sleep patterns are disturbed when his or her work shift is changed and how failing to get enough sleep night after night can put a person at risk for mistakes and accidents. The program describes research being done on sleep disorders such as sleep apnea and the many varieties of insomnia.

A large part of the video lesson is devoted to the important, though sometimes mysterious, topic of dreams and dreaming. Various theories about dreaming are examined, and there are accounts of research using state-of-the-art methods such as PET scans to reveal what goes on in the brain during dreaming.

As you watch the video program, consider the following questions:

1. What questions about the nature of sleep have been answered by modern science, and what important questions remain unanswered?

2. Is noted sleep researcher William Dement exaggerating or being literal when he says that "without sleep, we die"?

3. How do body rhythms influence one's ability to sleep?

4. What does Dement say about "sleep debt" and impaired performance?

5. How does Mark Rosekind describe his research on the stages of sleep?

6. What are some of the sleep disorders discussed by Dement and treated at Mark Stevenson's clinic?

7. What techniques and devices for dream research do Allan Hobson and Monte Buchsbaum describe?

8. What theories of the nature and function of dreaming are discussed?

9. What does Allan Hobson say about Freud's psychoanalytic theory of dream interpretation, and how does Hobson, one of the originators of the activation-synthesis theory, describe the dreaming process?

10. What can be learned from dreams, and how may dreams be controlled and/or made to serve waking purposes?

Review Exercises

Vocabulary Check

Match the following key terms and concepts with the appropriate definitions from the list below.

1. ___ altered state of consciousness (p. 160)

2. ___ biological rhythm (p. 140)

3. ___ circadian rhythm (p. 141; video)

4. ___ consciousness (p. 139)

5. ___ dissociation (p. 170)

6. ___ hypnosis (p. 168)

7. ___ infradian rhythm (p. 141)

8. ___ melatonin (p. 142)

9. ___ psychoactive drug (p. 161)

10. ___ rapid eye movement (REM) sleep (p. 150; video)

11. ___ seasonal affective disorder (SAD) (pp. 143–144)

12. ___ states of consciousness (p. 139)

13. ___ stimulants (p. 162)

14. ___ tolerance (p. 165)

15. ___ ultradian rhythm (p. 141)

a. increased resistance to a drug's effects with continued use

b. a periodic, more or less regular fluctuation in a biological system; may or may not have psychological implications

c. a condition, involving severe depression, whose symptoms occur every winter, when periods of daylight are short, and which clears up every spring, as daylight increases

d. a biological rhythm that occurs less frequently than once a day

e. drug capable of influencing perception, mood, cognition, or behavior

f. substances such as cocaine, amphetamines ("uppers"), nicotine, and caffeine that speed up activity in the central nervous system

g. the awareness of the environment and one's own existence, sensations, and thoughts

h. a biological rhythm with a period (from peak to peak or trough to trough) of about 24 hours

i. sleep periods characterized by eye movement, loss of muscle tone, and dreaming

j. a deliberately produced state of consciousness that differs from ordinary wakefulness or sleep

k. a biological rhythm that occurs more frequently than once a day

l. separation of consciousness into distinct parts

m. distinctive and discrete patterns in the functioning of consciousness, characterized by particular modes of perception, thought, memory, or feeling

n. a condition in which attention is focused and a person is extremely responsive to suggestion

o. a hormone secreted by the pineal gland; it is involved in the regulation of circadian rhythms

Other Key Terms and Concepts

activation-synthesis theory (p. 157; video)

alpha waves (p. 151)

delta waves (p. 151)

depressants (p. 162)

endogenous (p. 140)

entrainment (p. 140)

information-processing approach to dreams (p. 157)

insomnia (p. 174; video)

internal desynchronization (p. 142)

lucid dream (p. 153; video)

non-REM (NREM) sleep (p. 150; video)

opiates (p. 162)

premenstrual syndrome (PMS) (p. 145)

problem-focused approach to dreaming (p. 155)

psychedelic drugs (p. 162)

psychoanalytic theory of dreams (p. 154)

sleep apnea (p. 174; video)

sociocognitive explanation of hypnosis (pp. 171–172)

suprachiasmic nucleus (SCN) (p. 142)

withdrawal symptoms (p. 165)

Completion

Fill each blank with the most appropriate term from the list of answers below.

16. Internal _____, when circadian rhythms are thrown out of phase with one another, may be implicated in such accidents as Three Mile Island, Chernobyl, and the *Exxon Valdez* oil spill.

17. Some biological rhythms are associated with _____ or _____ changes, which makes them particularly interesting to psychologists.

18. Stage 3 and stage 4 sleep are characterized by the slow, regular _____ brain waves, whereas _____ waves are associated with relaxed wakefulness, rather than deep sleep.

19. The theory that most dreams are largely a matter of _____ contends that they reflect the ongoing emotional preoccupations of waking life.

20. According to the _____ theories, dreaming is a kind of mental housekeeping, during which the brain sorts old and new data into such categories as "wanted" and "unwanted."

21. According to the _____ theory, dreaming is the result of neurons firing spontaneously in the lower part of the brain, sending otherwise meaningless messages to the cortex, which tries to combine them with existing knowledge to make them coherent.

22. Psychoactive drugs, such as cocaine and amphetamines, that speed up activity in the central nervous system are called _____; _____, such as alcohol, tranquilizers, and barbiturates, are drugs that slow down activity in the central nervous system.

23. Each person's _____, including body weight, individual tolerance for a drug, and initial state of arousal, will influence his or her response to that drug at that time; so will his or her _____: the expectations about the drug's effects, the reasons for taking the drug, and the presence or absence of a desire to justify some behavior by being "under the influence."

24. Because people under its influence are in a heightened state of responsiveness to suggestions that may affect their perception, memory, and motivation, _____ has many applications in medicine and psychology.

25. According to Ernest Hilgard, hypnosis is an altered state of
_____ involving _____, in which one part of the mind
operates independently of another and may even function as a
_____ that watches but doesn't participate in the hypnosis.

activation-synthesis   dissociation   mental

alpha   emotional   mental set

consciousness   hidden observer   physical condition

delta   hypnosis   problem solving

depressants   information-processing   stimulants

desynchronization

True-False

Read the following statements carefully and mark each true (T) or false (F).

26. ___ The female menstrual cycle, which occurs on average every 28 days, is an example of an infradian rhythm.

27. ___ The most frequently studied circadian rhythms are the cycles occurring during sleep.

28. ___ People seldom dream during REM sleep.

29. ___ There is still considerable debate on the purpose of REM sleep.

30. ___ No one has ever figured out how to control the action in dreams.

31. ___ According to the psychoanalytic explanation, dreams are exactly what they seem to be: absurd fantasies without meaning or logic.

32. ___ Many psychologists believe that most dreams reflect the ongoing emotional preoccupations of waking life, such as concern over relationships, work, sex, or health.

33. ___ The activation-synthesis theory of dreaming originated in the time of Shakespeare.

34. ___ Animal studies suggest that repeated use of certain psychoactive drugs causes permanent brain damage.

35. ___ Opiates are solely street drugs and have no legitimate uses.

36. ___ The many scientific studies of marijuana use have produced a consensus about the drug's effects and dangers.

37. ___ The environmental setting in which an individual uses a drug has little or no influence on his or her response to that drug.

38. ___ Brain waves during hypnosis are more like those produced during sleep than those of ordinary wakefulness.

39. ___ Psychologists who study hypnosis can gain new insights into human suggestibility, perception, memory, motivation, and the power of imagination.

Short-Answer Questions

As a final review exercise, write brief answers to demonstrate that you are achieving the learning objectives of this lesson.

1. Define and provide examples of biological rhythms, and explain why psychologists are interested in studying them.

2. Describe REM sleep and the four stages of non-REM sleep, and explain the pattern of the sleep cycle.

3. Discuss dreaming and the major explanations of why we dream: the psychoanalytic explanation, dreams as problem solving, dreams as information processing, and the activation-synthesis theory.

4. Discuss the common effects of psychoactive drugs and the results of abusing or being addicted to stimulant, depressant, opiate, and psychedelic drugs.

5. Explain how physical condition, past usage of a drug, mental set, and environmental setting can affect an individual's response to a drug.

6. Describe the general nature of hypnosis and provide examples of how hypnosis is used in medicine and psychology.

Self-Test

1. A circadian rhythm is a biological cycle that occurs
   a. approximately every 24 hours.
   b. more frequently than once a day.
   c. less frequently than once a day.
   d. in response to seasonal changes.

2. The hormone _____, secreted by the pineal gland, may play a role in synchronizing the brain with the natural environment's light-dark cycle.
   a. epinephrine
   b. norepinephrine
   c. estrogen
   d. melatonin

3. _____ is an example of internal desynchronization, when circadian rhythms are thrown out of phase with one another because a person's normal routine changes.
   a. Adolescence
   b. Premenstrual syndrome
   c. Jet lag
   d. Seasonal affective disorder (SAD)

4. People tend to be hardest to arouse during
   a. stage 1 sleep.
   b. stage 2 sleep.
   c. stage 3 sleep.
   d. stage 4 sleep.

5. In human beings, _____ of the periods of dreaming are likely to be associated with rapid eye movement (REM).
   a. none
   b. all
   c. most
   d. few

6. The stages of deep sleep
   a. occur fairly consistently throughout the night.
   b. become less frequent or disappear as morning approaches.
   c. become more frequent as morning approaches.
   d. coincide with periods of REM sleep.

7. So-called lucid dreams, in which you know you are dreaming and feel as though you are conscious, may be attributable to a split in consciousness known as
   a. multiple personality.
   b. dissociation.
   c. fragmentation.
   d. delusion.

8. In Sigmund Freud's psychoanalytic explanation of dreams, he contended that to understand a dream, we must distinguish its _____ from its _____.
   a. unconscious meaning; conscious meaning
   b. sexual symbols; actual content
   c. symbolic content; hidden content
   d. manifest content; latent content

9. According to the theory that sees dreams as problem solving, the symbols and metaphors in a dream
   a. convey the dream's true meaning.
   b. disguise the dream's true meaning.
   c. are imaginary constructs created after the dreamer awakens.
   d. are always filled with sexual meaning.

10. Which of the following explanations of why we dream theorizes that during sleep and dreaming the brain assimilates new data and updates data already stored in memory?
    a. psychoanalytic explanation
    b. information-processing approaches
    c. activation-synthesis theory
    d. dreams as problem solving theory

11. Which of the following is an explanation of dreaming based on the study of biological processes, such as the firing of neurons in the brain?

    a. psychoanalytic explanation

    b. information-processing approaches

    c. activation-synthesis theory

    d. the REM sleep model

12. Substances that can influence perception, mood, memory, cognition, or behavior are known as _____

    a. addictive

    b. illegal

    c. psychedelic

    d. psychoactive

13. Alcohol, tranquilizers, barbiturates, and other drugs known as sedatives or hypnotics, which slow down the activity in the central nervous system, fall into the category of

    a. stimulants.

    b. depressants.

    c. psychedelic drugs.

    d. opiates.

14. Which category of drugs relieves pain, mimicking the action of endorphins (naturally occurring neuromodulators capable of suppressing pain perception in the brain)?

    a. stimulants

    b. depressants

    c. psychedelic drugs

    d. opiates

15. Abuse of/addiction to which of the following substances can result in blackouts, liver damage, mental and neurological impairment, psychosis, and possibly death?

    a. heroin

    b. cocaine

    c. alcohol

    d. marijuana

16. Although no firm conclusions have yet been drawn about either the physical or psychological effects of the nonmedical use of _____ numerous negative effects have been reported, including heart and liver disease, decreased testicular size, aggression, anxiety, and even psychosis.

    a. marijuana

    b. barbiturates

    c. anabolic steroids

    d. amphetamines

17. Which of the following is LEAST likely to influence the effect of a given drug on the individual using it?

    a. that person's physical condition

    b. the fact that many other people use the drug

    c. the fact that the person has used the drug before

    d. what the person expects the drug to do

18. In studies in which some subjects drank vodka and tonic and others unknowingly drank just tonic and lime juice, those who only *thought* they'd been drinking liquor still exhibited some behavior associated with the effects of alcohol. The results of such studies may be attributable to which of the following?

    a. physical condition

    b. experience with the drug

    c. mental set

    d. environmental setting

19. Which of the following probably accounts most for the fact that the same person who gets drowsy after one beer or glass of wine remain alert?

    a. physical condition

    b. experience with the drug

    c. mental set

    d. environmental setting

20. According to noted authority Ernest Hilgard, hypnosis is

    a. a form of sleep.

    b. an illusion produced by the hypnotized subject's desire to please the hypnotist.

    c. an altered or split state of consciousness.

    d. a mechanism for gaining access to a person's real feelings and true personality.

21. Regarding the use of "hypnotically refreshed" testimony in court cases, both the American Medical Association (AMA) and the American Psychological Association (APA) are on record as

    a. supporting its use, because hypnosis can encourage vivid imagery that might prompt a witness to recall critical facts, such as license numbers.

    b. opposing its use, because pseudomemories and errors are so common in hypnotically induced recall.

    c. opposing its use unless the evidence in question was obtained by a member of one of their organizations.

    d. refusing to testify in cases using such evidence.

22. Whatever hypnosis is, by studying it, psychologists are learning much about each of the following EXCEPT

    a. human suggestibility.

    b. the power of imagination.

    c. the way we perceive the present and remember the past.

    d. individuals' past lives or abduction by aliens, as revealed in hypnotically refreshed accounts.

Study Activities

The following activity challenges you to use your critical thinking and demonstrate how what you are learning can be applied to you and your own life. Try this activity and/or those your instructor assigns.

Learn more about how drugs touch your personal life and affect the society in which you live. In an era when entire nations are fighting "wars" against drugs or having drug traffickers declare war on them, it hardly seems necessary to ask students to increase their awareness of consciousness-altering substances. But the problems of drug abuse and addiction seem to be getting worse, not better, so the more you know about the subject, the greater the likelihood that you will be able to cope successfully with the challenges these problems present. Moreover, not all uses of drugs pose problems. You should also be aware that the role of drugs in medical treatment programs continues to grow as new substances and approaches are developed to deal with physical disorders. Similarly, you should know how significant psychoactive drugs are in the treatment of emotional disorders.

Approach this study activity from two directions. First, do some systematic research into the latest findings on what drugs can do. Use the bibliography in the textbook to pinpoint some recent works on the topic. Look into both drug abuse and pharmacology. Try to discover what the latest research says about which drugs are the most dangerous, and in what ways. Check into the promise and potential dangers of science devising entirely new substances. Work at getting the latest and most authoritative information.

Next, do some personal research. Use yourself, your family, and your friends as subjects of an informal survey on drug use. This shouldn't be thought of as an exposé of bad habits, but rather as a nonjudgmental inquiry into how big a part drugs play in ordinary people's lives. For example, ask under what circumstances and how often you and others take over-the-counter medication. Ask how many and what kinds of prescription drugs are taken regularly. Your relationship with the people you survey will determine whether or not you ask them about the use of commonly abused drugs. In many cases, you won't even have to ask. If you know the people well (including yourself), you will know who drinks heavily or uses street drugs, and you will know who has had family, school, employment, financial, medical, legal, or other problems as a result of the use of consciousness-altering substances.

After you have compiled information from both your formal research and your informal survey, notice where the information from one overlaps the data from the other. You should be able to test the reliability and validity of your survey against what the experts have said; at the same time, your personal survey should supply real-world examples of the conclusions drawn by the trained researchers.

Lesson 6

Sensation and Perception

Assignments

For the most systematic coverage of this lesson, we suggest that you complete the assignments in the sequence listed below.

Before viewing the video program:

- Read the "Learning Objectives" and "Overview" for this lesson. Use the Learning Objectives to guide your reading, viewing, and thinking.

- Read the "Viewing Notes" for this lesson.

- Read Chapter 6, "Sensation and Perception," in the Wade and Tavris text. First, familiarize yourself with its contents by reading the Chapter Outline. As you read, note terms and concepts set in bold or italic type, especially those defined in the margins.

View the video program, "Sensation and Perception"

After viewing the video program:

- Briefly note your answers to the questions at the end of the "Viewing Notes."

- Review all reading assignments for this lesson, including the Summary at the end of Chapter 6 in the textbook.

- Complete the "Review Exercises" to strengthen your understanding of this lesson's central concepts and terminology. Pay special attention to the "Vocabulary Check" exercise and the additional terms and concepts that follow—page references indicate where in the text assignment each term is defined. [Remember: there is a complete Glossary at the end of the text.]

- Take the "Self-Test" to measure the degree to which you are achieving this lesson's learning objectives. Check your answers against the "Answer Key" and review when necessary.

- Follow the suggestions in the "Study Activities" section at the end of this lesson and complete any other activities and projects assigned by your instructor.

Learning Objectives

When you have completed all assignments in this lesson, you should be able to:

1. Distinguish between sensation and perception, and explain the interrelationship between them.

2. Describe how human beings extract information from the environment and organize it into perceptions.

3. Define and explain sensory adaptation, selective attention, and sensory deprivation. Identify these processes in real-life situations.

4. Describe the structure and functions of each of the sensory systems: vision, hearing, taste, smell, skin senses, kinesthesis, and sense of balance.

5. Describe human perceptual powers and explain perceptual constancy and illusion, giving examples of each.

6. Explain how a person's needs, beliefs, emotions, and expectations can influence his or her perceptions, and define the relationship between inborn perceptual abilities and environmental experience and learning.

7. Explain why the history of research on psychic phenomena has been one of initial enthusiasm followed by disappointment.

Overview

Much of what psychologists know about how and why people learn, think, and act as they do is based upon knowledge of human sensation and perception. This lesson defines these central concepts and explains their critically important interrelationship. The text and video program clarify the often complex processes by which the human sensory system detects and encodes information from the environment or from internal events and transmits it to the brain to be analyzed and organized into perceptions. The lesson introduces **psychophysics** and concepts such as **absolute threshold**, **difference threshold**, **sensory adaptation**, **sensory deprivation**, and **selective attention**.

The lesson describes the structure and functions of the sensory systems: **vision, hearing, taste, smell**, the **skin senses, kinesthesis**, and the **sense of balance**. The text provides detailed explanations of how each system works, and the video program offers several graphic examples of sensory processes, with special attention to visual perception and the perception of pain. Because human beings rely so much on vision, a large part of the lesson is devoted to the workings of the visual system, from the constituent parts of the eye to the problems of repairing childhood strabismus (misaligned eyes) before it disrupts the brain's ability to handle the child's visual input. The subject of pain is explored, including discussion of the **gate-control theory** of pain, the role of chemical substances released at the site of damaged tissue, and the impact of endorphins—the brain's natural painkillers.

Human perceptual powers are examined, including innate and learned perceptual abilities, conscious and nonconscious perception, subliminal perception, division of the world into meaningful perceptual units and patterns, and the location of objects in space. **Perceptual constancies**, **illusions**, and psychological and cultural influences on perception are also discussed.

Both the text and video explore how psychological factors such as needs, beliefs, memories, emotions, and expectations influence perception. The text shows why so-called extrasensory perception (ESP) seems to be more attributable to such psychological factors than to physical forces and mechanisms. The lesson explains that what we perceive involves the interplay of raw sensory data and the brain's powers of interpretation and organization. The lesson considers the relationship between innate perceptual abilities and what is learned or experienced.

Viewing Notes

This video program explains how we construct reality from raw material provided by our senses and interpreted and organized into meaningful patterns by our brains. It points out that the reality we perceive is filtered because our senses are limited in many ways. Moreover, when our brains process sensory input to create our perceptions, the result is not an absolute "reality" shared by other creatures experiencing the same thing, but a kind of code. Calling something red or blue or hot or cold, for example, reflects our own model of the real world. In the video, experts explain the complex sensory and perceptual process.

Because human beings rely so heavily on sight, the program pays considerable attention to human vision. There are enlightening demonstrations of how the eye works, how the brain processes visual information, how various visual cues make our vision more accurate and effective, and how medical science is dealing with some of the problems people can have with their eyes and their vision.

The video program describes the strategies the brain uses to process sensations into perceptions, demonstrating the influence of expectations and emotional states on perception. The role that illusions and misperceptions can play in real-world situations is examined, and there is a segment on the biological and psychological factors at work in the perception and inhibition of pain.

As you watch the video program, consider the following questions:

1. What is the relationship between reality and human perception, as explained by Jack Yellott?

2. How does Ernest Greene explain visual perception?

3. Why is binocular vision important to humans, and what does Yellott say about some of the cues that aid visual perception?

4. What does David Van Essen say about how the eye and the brain turn sensory stimuli into visual perception?

5. What do Kenneth Wright and Barbara Fox say about how children develop or achieve normal vision?

6. How does Yellott explain that the form a percept (an impression of an object obtained through the senses and received by the brain) finally takes is determined by the interplay between raw sensory data and the brain's interpretive mechanism?

7. What do illusions and misperceptions tell us about how our perceptual system works?

8. What do John Liebeskind and Ronald Young say about how the human pain-inhibiting system works?

Review Exercises

Vocabulary Check

Match the following key terms and concepts with the appropriate definitions from the list below.

1. ___ absolute threshold (p. 182)

2. ___ difference threshold (p. 183)

3. ___ gate-control theory (p. 209; video)

4. ___ gustation (p. 204)

5. ___ kinesthesis (p. 210)

6. ___ monocular cues (p. 196; video)

7. ___ olfaction (p. 206)

8. ___ parapsychology (p. 218)

9. ___ perception (p. 180)

10. ___ perceptual constancy (p. 197)

11. ___ perceptual illusion (p. 198; video)

12. ___ selective attention (p. 187)

13. ___ sensation (p. 180)

14. ___ sensory adaptation (p. 185)

15. ___ sensory deprivation (p. 186)

a. the smallest difference in stimulation that can be reliably detected by an observer when two stimuli are compared; also called the just noticeable difference (jnd)

b. the sense of smell

c. the process by which the brain organizes and interprets sensory information

d. absence of normal levels of sensory stimulation

e. the detection of physical energy emitted or reflected by physical objects; it occurs when energy in the external environment or the body stimulates receptors in the sense organs

f. the accurate perception of objects as stable or unchanged despite changes in the sensory patterns they produce

g. the study of purported psychic phenomena such as ESP and mental telepathy

h. the reduction or disappearance of sensory responsiveness that occurs when stimulation is unchanging and repetitious

i. the theory that the experience of pain depends in part on whether pain impulses get past a neurological "gate" and thus reach the brain

j. the smallest quantity of physical energy that can be reliably detected by an observer

k. the sense of taste

l. visual cues, such as interposition and linear perspective, , which do not depend on using both eyes

m. an erroneous or misleading perception of reality

n. the sense of body position and movement of body parts

o. focusing attention on selected aspects of the environment and blocking out others

Other Key Terms and Concepts

audition (p. 200)

binocular cues (p. 196; video)

brightness (p. 188)

cochlea (p. 202)

complexity of light (p. 188)

cones (p. 189)

convergence (p. 196)

dark adaptation (p. 190)

doctrine of specific nerve energies (p. 181)

equilibrium (p. 210)

extrasensory perception (ESP) (pp. 217–219)

feature detectors (p. 190)

frequency (of sound wave) (p. 201)

ganglion cells (p. 190)

Gestalt principles (p. 195)

hue (p. 188)

loudness (p. 200)

neuromatrix theory (p. 209)

opponent-process theory (p. 193)

papillae (p. 204)

perceptual set (p. 214)

pheromones (p. 207)

pitch (p. 201)

psychophysics (p. 182)

retina (p. 189; video)

retinal disparity (p. 196)

rods (p. 189)

saturation (p. 188)

semicircular canals (p. 210)

sense organs (p. 179)

sense receptors (p. 180)

signal-detection theory (p. 184)

subliminal perception (p. 215)

taste buds (p. 204)

timbre (p. 201)

trichromatic theory (p. 192)

Completion

Fill each blank with the most appropriate term from the list of answers below.

16. Sense _____ are parts of the body that contain the sense _____.

17. Sensation depends on a process called _____, which converts sensory stimuli into electrical nerve impulses that can be interpreted by the brain.

18. The psychophysical theory that divides detection of a sensory signal into a sensory process and a decision process is called the _____ theory.

19. The capacity for _____ frees the brain from having to respond to everything the sensory receptors transmit to it.

20. The _____ (the membrane lining the back of the interior of the eyeball) contains the _____, visual receptors that respond especially well to dim light but aren't involved in color vision, and the _____, the receptors involved in color vision.

21. Three dimensions of the auditory experience are _____, _____, and _____.

22. A person walking toward you from a distance does not seem to "grow" as he or she gets closer because your visual system possesses a capacity for _____.

23. A habitual way of perceiving, based on expectations, is called a _____.

24. Although much of perception is innate, _____ and learning influence the development of perceptual skills.

25. Seeing and responding to a message that is below the absolute threshold to be consciously seen is described as _____.

cones	perceptual set	selective attention
culture	pitch	signal detection
loudness	receptors	subliminal perception
organs	retina	timbre
perceptual constancy	rods	transduction

True-False

Read the following statements carefully and mark each true (T) or false (F).

26. ___ Sensation is the process by which sensory impulses are organized and interpreted.

27. ___ Human vision is sufficiently sensitive to detect a candle flame from 30 miles on a clear night.

28. ___ You will stop noticing an unchanging, repetitious stimulus—such as a sound or smell—because your sensory receptors have temporarily stopped responding.

29. ___ Neither rods nor cones are sensitive enough to detect pheromones.

30. ___ The cochlea is an organ central to the sense of smell.

31. ___ The sense of smell is more important to human beings than to most animals.

32. ___ The gate-control theory describes the process of selective attention whereby unwanted sensory stimuli are not allowed beyond the "gate" in the spinal cord.

33. ___ Research indicates that certain basic perceptual processes are nonconscious—they occur outside of awareness.

34. ___ Perceptual constancy refers to your readiness to perceive a stimulus in a particular, habitual way.

35. ___ Because illusions are random and unpredictable perceptual errors, they are of little value or interest to psychologists studying the systematic characteristics of the perceptual system.

36. ___ Perception is too thoroughly programmed biologically to be influenced by what an individual desires, thinks, feels, or expects.

37. ___ Gestalt psychologists believe that the strategies the human brain uses to organize and experience the world as whole patterns or configurations involve grouping sensory building blocks into perceptual units such as proximity, closure, similarity, and continuity.

38. ___ Subliminal persuasion, using such techniques as flashing subliminal slogans on television or slipping subliminal images into magazine ads, has proved so effective that few advertisers risk promoting their products these days without employing this powerful marketing device.

Short-Answer Questions

As a final review exercise, write brief answers to demonstrate that you are achieving the learning objectives of this lesson.

1. Distinguish between sensation and perception, and explain the interrelationship between them.

2. Describe how human beings extract information from the environment and organize it into perceptions.

3. Define and explain sensory adaptation, selective attention, and sensory deprivation. Identify these processes in real-life situations.

4. Describe the structure and functions of each of the sensory systems: vision, hearing, taste, smell, skin senses, kinesthesis, and sense of balance.

5. Describe human perceptual powers and explain perceptual constancy and illusion, giving examples of each.

6. Explain how a person's needs, beliefs, emotions, and expectations can influence his or her perceptions, and define the relationship between inborn perceptual abilities and environmental experience and learning.

7. Explain why the history of research on psychic phenomena has been one of initial enthusiasm followed by disappointment.

Self-Test

1. The detection of physical energy emitted or reflected by physical objects; it occurs when energy in the external environment or the body stimulates receptors in the sense organs

   a. cognition.

   b. sensation.

   c. perception.

   d. adaptation.

2. The _____ are specialized cells that convert physical energy in the environment into electrical energy that can be transmitted as nerve impulses to the brain.

   a. threshold cells

   b. ganglion cells

   c. sense organs

   d. sense receptors

3. Psychologists study _____ and _____ because they are the foundation of learning, thinking, and acting.

   a. transduction; audition

   b. perception; olfaction

   c. sensation; perception

   d. sensation; selective attention

4. All human senses evolved for the same purpose: to

   a. increase our ability to enjoy the environment.

   b. make us more aware of our feelings and internal states.

   c. provide information that could improve our ability to communicate.

   d. help us survive.

5. To say "the sky is blue, the grass is green, and a rose is red" is to describe

   a. reality.

   b. the role of the human brain in deciding on information sent by sense receptors.

   c. each thing's chemical composition.

   d. what all normal humans and other species capable of perception actually see.

6. The _____ is a stimulus that probably would **NOT** trigger sensory adaptation.

   a. sound of a dripping faucet

   b. feel on your skin of a chair upholstered in a rough fabric

   c. taste of a spicy meal

   d. smell of spilled ammonia

7. The central finding of sensory deprivation experiments seems to be that

   a. without sensory input, people go insane.

   b. the human brain has trouble functioning normally without a certain amount of sensory stimulation during daily life.

   c. anyone protected from sensory stimulation is sure to be more relaxed, confident, and creative.

   d. it is difficult to get sufficient numbers of people to volunteer to be experimental subjects.

8. When you are at a big party and are part of a particular conversation, the reason you don't really hear all the other conversations around you, or the music and other party sounds, is because of

   a. sensory adaptation.

   b. sensory deprivation.

   c. selective attention.

   d. perceptual constancy.

9. Which of the following is **NOT** a dimension of the visual experience?

    a. timbre

    b. hue

    c. brightness

    d. saturation

10. Which of the following is **NOT** a dimension of the auditory experience?

    a. loudness

    b. pitch

    c. saturation

    d. timbre

11. Taste, or gustation, occurs because chemicals stimulate receptors in the mouth that detect four basic tastes:

    a. sweet, sour, fresh, and rancid.

    b. salty, sour, bitter, and sweet.

    c. cold, hot, moist, and dry.

    d. spicy, mild, sweet, and sour.

12. _____ tells us where our body parts are located and lets us know when they move.

    a. Equilibrium

    b. Olfaction

    c. Kinesthesis

    d. Subliminal perception

13. A person who has lost an arm or leg may sometimes experience so-called phantom pain in the missing limb; this phenomenon can be explained by

    a. kinesthesia.

    b. the neuromatrix theory.

    c. the trichromatic theory.

    d. the difference threshold.

14. Although perceptual illusions—erroneous or misleading perceptions of reality—can occur in any sensory modality, _____ illusions have been studied more than other kinds.

    a. auditory

    b. visual

    c. olfactory

    d. gustatory

15. The best-studied perceptual constancies include

    a. brightness, focus, and angle.

    b. shape, location, and size.

    c. color, texture, and content.

    d. size, age, and weight.

16. Research findings on subliminal perception

    a. prove that such a nonconscious perceptual process doesn't actually exist.

    b. are potentially important for theories of how the mind works.

    c. are suspect because they seldom derive from double-blind studies.

    d. are uniformly supportive of the claims that subliminal messages are irresistible influences on consumers and voters.

17. Perhaps the most important difference between the way a camera captures a scene and the way a human perceives the same scene is that

    a. film can be made far more sensitive than the human retina.

    b. cameras can have zoom lenses.

    c. human vision makes no permanent record like a photograph or slide.

    d. human thoughts and feelings can influence perception.

18. Because previous experience gives us certain expectations, we may be ready to perceive a stimulus in a particular way. This habitual way of perceiving is called

    a. selective attention.

    b. a perceptual set.

    c. perceptual constancy.

    d. sensory adaptation.

19. The perceptual abilities of human children are

    a. innate; each child is born with exactly what he or she will need to perceive the world.

    b. entirely learned and trained throughout life.

    c. largely inborn, but improve throughout childhood.

    d. identical to those of adults.

20. Much of the evidence for extrasensory perception comes from

    a. replicated scientific studies.

    b. anecdotal accounts.

    c. hypnotically refreshed memories.

    d. the testimony of people who have been abducted by aliens.

21. Which of the following is **NOT** true of the field of parapsychology?

    a. Researchers have extensively studied extrasensory perception.

    b. The existence of parapsychological (extrasensory) phenomena has been scientifically proved.

    c. Despite the failure of parapsychologists to find scientific evidence for ESP, about half of all Americans say they believe in it.

    d. Parapsychological research, employing improved methods, continues.

Study Activities

The following activity challenges you to use your critical thinking and demonstrate how what you are learning can be applied to you and your own life. Try this activity and/or those your instructor assigns.

The reading assignment for this lesson in the Wade and Tavris text (page 213) makes a provocative assertion that "because we human beings care about what we see, hear, taste, smell, and feel, psychological factors [such as needs, beliefs, emotions, and expectations] can influence what we perceive and how we perceive it." The purpose of this study activity is to determine if this assertion holds true in your experience, to see if it might even apply to you and your perceptions.

Can you give examples of situations in which observers seemed to have different—even utterly contradictory—perceptions of the same event? Consider sporting events you have attended, seen on television, or in which you have participated. Have you ever noticed that umpires and referees make more wrong calls against you or the team you want to win? Have you seen athletes, particularly professional tennis players, who rage against calls that go against them, even when they couldn't possibly have seen what happened as clearly as the officials they curse for being wrong (and when most spectators could see the officials were right)? If you've seen, and especially if you've had such experiences, doesn't it seem that those having such one-sided perceptions—because they want and need their side to win—are sincerely convinced that their perceptions are correct?

On a more serious level, don't people in wartime usually see their adversaries as inhuman monsters who deserve to be destroyed? Similarly, don't different people perceive the same news event differently? Weren't people's opinions of what they saw happening in the video of the Rodney King beating by Los Angeles police officers affected by their feelings about the police in general or by their race or socioeconomic situation? If you saw the King video, the trial of the officers, and the Los Angeles riots that followed the not-guilty verdict, examine your perceptions. Being as objective as possible, think about whether anything you perceived was influenced by emotions, beliefs, and expectations you had before you witnessed these shocking events.

As a more formal exercise, for as many weeks as it takes to compile some informative data, keep a notebook handy and record what appear to be perceptions influenced by needs, beliefs, emotions, and expectations. Monitor news reports of clashes between people holding strong opinions on inflammatory issues such as abortion, the environment, prayer in schools, welfare, taxes and how they are used by government—anything that involves people with different perceptions of the same "facts." Note the details of ethnic, religious, political, and nationalistic clashes in places such as the former Soviet Union and Yugoslavia, the Middle East, Northern Ireland—and in the United States between citizens who resist government power and officials who exercise it. Watch for the "us-them" aspects of reasoning used to explain or justify acts that to you may appear irrational or obviously unjust.

Look for news accounts (even read some checkout-stand periodicals) of miraculous cures or manifestations, paranormal occurrences, UFO sightings, and the like. Don't forget to consider stories about legal cases, in which contradictory testimony by different individuals seems attributable to psychological predispositions the witnesses had before testifying—even before witnessing the events. The O. J. Simpson case was an obvious example.

Keep your record of anything that involves reports of events or encounters whose objectivity you can question by citing needs, beliefs, emotions, and expectations that may have influenced what the perceivers claim to have perceived. Don't forget to make notations of your own perceptions. When you watch a sports event, be aware of characterizing your team as right even when you have only your feelings and no real evidence for what you may honestly perceive.

Remember: The issue is not that people don't actually perceive what they claim to; it is that what they perceive is shaped by psychological influences of which they may not even be aware. This exercise should help you sharpen your awareness of how this pervasive and potentially disruptive process operates.

Learning

Assignments

For the most systematic coverage of this lesson, we suggest that you complete the assignments in the sequence listed below.

Before viewing the video program:

- Read the "Learning Objectives" and "Overview" for this lesson. Use the Learning Objectives to guide your reading, viewing, and thinking.

- Read the "Viewing Notes" for this lesson.

- Read Chapter 7, "Learning and Conditioning," in the Wade and Tavris text. First, familiarize yourself with its contents by reading the Chapter Outline. As you read, note terms and concepts set in bold or italic type, especially those defined in the margins.

View the video program, "Learning"

After viewing the video program:

- Briefly note your answers to the questions at the end of the "Viewing Notes."

- Review all reading assignments for this lesson, including the Summary at the end of Chapter 7 in the textbook.

- Complete the "Review Exercises" to strengthen your understanding of this lesson's central concepts and terminology. Pay special attention to the "Vocabulary Check" exercise and the additional terms and concepts that follow—page references indicate where in the text assignment each term is defined. [Remember: there is a complete Glossary at the end of the text.]

- Take the "Self-Test" to measure the degree to which you are achieving this lesson's learning objectives. Check your answers against the "Answer Key" and review when necessary.

- Follow the suggestions in the "Study Activities" section at the end of this lesson and complete any other activities and projects assigned by your instructor.

Learning Objectives

When you have completed all assignments in this lesson, you should be able to:

1. Describe the process of classical (Pavlovian) conditioning and apply the principles in real-life situations.

2. Describe the process of operant conditioning and explain how the basic types of behavioral consequences affect learning.

3. Compare the effects of continuous reinforcement and intermittent schedules of reinforcement on learning.

4. Discuss several potential disadvantages of using punishment in real-world situations.

5. Define behavior modification and discuss its uses.

6. Explain how the modification of behavior can be complicated by such factors as the impact of intrinsic and extrinsic reinforcers and the biological constraints on learning.

7. Describe kinds of learning (e.g., latent learning and observational learning) that pose some problems for traditional conditioning theories and may require mentalistic explanations.

8. Distinguish between behavioral and cognitive explanations of behavior, and discuss why many psychologists consider both approaches when dealing with real-world problems.

Overview

This lesson begins with a brief introduction to the psychological definition of learning, which is any relatively permanent change in behavior (or behavioral potential) that occurs as a result of experience. It covers the fundamental principles of **behaviorism**, which was the predominant influence on psychology as a whole throughout the 1950s and 1960s and remains one of the major perspectives in psychology.

The text assignment and video program introduce **classical (Pavlovian) conditioning** and **operant conditioning** and describe some of their real-life applications. Pavlov's famous conditioning experiments with salivating dogs are described, and the role and relationship of **stimuli** and **responses** are explained. The coverage of operant conditioning includes a video interview with B. F. Skinner, who is universally acknowledged as the foremost proponent of operant principles. In what was one of the last interviews of his life, he personally defines operant conditioning and its behavioral consequences.

Types of **reinforcement** and **schedules of reinforcement** are compared, and the potential disadvantages of **punishment** in real-world situations are examined. The uses of **behavior modification** are explored in the text. Token economy, a form of behavior modification, is included in a particularly illuminating segment of the video. The lesson explains how the modification of behavior can be complicated by such factors as the interaction of **extrinsic** and **intrinsic reinforcers** and by the **biological constraints on learning**.

Kinds of learning (such as **latent learning** and **observational learning**) that pose some problems for traditional conditioning theories are discussed. Behavioral and cognitive explanations of behavior are differentiated, and it is shown that both can be employed in dealing with real-world problems.

Viewing Notes

The video program "Learning" focuses on the fundamental processes of classical (Pavlovian) conditioning and operant conditioning and on the real-world applications of behavioral psychology. The program explains how conditioning provides a scientific basis for learning. The basic principles are introduced and explained, and their major uses are described. One segment of the video lesson is an interview with B. F. Skinner, the most noted figure in behaviorism and the person most often identified with operant conditioning. This interview was conducted just for this telecourse, shortly before Skinner's death. Another major segment of the video program was shot at a child-development center where the principles of operant conditioning are used to help so-called hyperactive children whose severe behavior and learning problems result from attention disorders.

As you watch the video program, consider the following questions:

1. How do John Garcia and Carl Gustaveson make practical use of classical conditioning to deal humanely with coyotes who preyed on farmers' livestock?

2. How do classical conditioning principles help cancer patients receiving chemotherapy?

3. How does B. F. Skinner define and describe operant conditioning?

4. How were the lives of some of the people in the video lesson changed by operant conditioning?

5. What does operant conditioning teach us about the training of dogs?

6. How does the University of California at Irvine Development Center use behavior modification techniques in its programs?

7. What role has a token economy played in the Irvine Center's success?

8. How is cognitive psychology brought into play at the Irvine Center?

9. How are the methods used at the Irvine Center applied when the children are at home?

Review Exercises

Vocabulary Check

Match the following key terms and concepts with the appropriate definitions from the list below.

1. ___ behavior modification (p. 247; video)

2. ___ conditioned stimulus (CS) (p. 228; video)

3. ___ extinction (pp. 228, 241; video)

4. ___ instinctive drift (p. 244)

5. ___ intermittent (partial) schedule of reinforcement (p. 241)

6. ___ intrinsic reinforcers (p. 251)

7. ___ latent learning (p. 256)

8. ___ learning (p. 226)

9. ___ negative reinforcement (p. 238)

10. ___ operant conditioning (p. 236; video)

11. ___ primary reinforcer (p. 238)

12. ___ punishment (p. 237)

13. ___ reinforcement (p. 237; video)

14. ___ token economy (video)

a. a relatively permanent change in behavior (or behavioral potential) due to experience

b. the weakening and eventual disappearance of a learned response

c. a reinforcement procedure in which a response is followed by the removal, delay, or decrease in intensity of an unpleasant stimulus; as a result, the response becomes stronger or more likely to occur

d. the classical conditioning term for an initially neutral stimulus that comes to elicit a conditioned response after being associated with an unconditioned stimulus

e. the application of conditioning techniques to reduce or eliminate maladaptive or problematic behavior or to teach new responses

f. the process by which a response becomes more or less likely to occur, depending upon its consequences

g. any stimulus or event that reduces the probability that the response it follows will recur

h. reinforcers that are by their very nature related to the activity being reinforced

i. a reinforcement schedule in which a particular response is sometimes, but not always, reinforced

j. the tendency of an organism to revert to an instinctive behavior over time, which can place a biological constraint on learning

k. a behavior modification technique in which secondary reinforcers are used as reinforcers and can eventually be exchanged for primary or other secondary reinforcers

l. a stimulus that is inherently reinforcing, typically satisfying a physiological need; food, for example

m. the process by which a stimulus strengthens or increases the probability of the response that it follows

n. a form of learning not immediately expressed in an overt response; occurs without obvious reinforcement

Other Key Terms and Concepts

behaviorism (p. 226)

biological limits on learning (p. 244)

classical (Pavlovian) conditioning (p. 228; video)

conditioned response (CR) (p. 228; video)

continuous reinforcement (p. 241)

counterconditioning (p. 233)

discriminative stimulus (p. 241)

extrinsic reinforcers (p. 251)

fixed-interval schedule (p. 243)

fixed-ratio schedule (p. 242)

higher-order conditioning (p. 229)

law of effect (video)

observational learning (p. 254)

phobia (p. 233)

positive reinforcement (p. 238)

primary punisher (p. 238)

schedules of reinforcement (pp. 241–243; video)

secondary punisher (p. 238)

secondary reinforcer (p. 238)

shaping (p. 243)

Skinner box (p. 240)

social-cognitive theories (pp. 253–254)

spontaneous recovery (p. 229)

stimulus discrimination (pp. 230, 241; video)

stimulus generalization (pp. 229, 241)

successive approximations (p. 244)

unconditioned response (UR) (p. 227; video)

unconditioned stimulus (US) (p. 227; video)

variable-interval schedule (p. 243)

variable-ratio schedule (p. 242)

Completion

Fill each blank with the most appropriate term from the list of answers below.

15. Classical, or _____, conditioning is the process by which a previously neutral stimulus acquires the capacity to elicit a response through association with a stimulus that naturally elicits a similar response.

16. If you train a dog to salivate at the sound of a bell by giving it food each time you ring the bell and then you ring the bell without presenting the food, the dog's salivation response will weaken and eventually disappear and _____ will have occurred.

17. B. F. Skinner is the person most closely associated with _____ conditioning.

18. A stimulus or event that strengthens or increases the probability of the response that follows is called a _____.

19. If a response is sometimes, but not always, reinforced, the reinforcement is on an _____, or partial, schedule.

20. Real-world studies show that _____ has some serious disadvantages as a method of behavior control.

21. The application of operant conditioning techniques (and some classical ones) in real-world settings is called _____.

22. Many behavior modification programs rely on a feature known as a _____, in which secondary reinforcers are used to modify behavior and can later be exchanged for primary reinforcers, such as food or candy, or for other secondary reinforcers.

23. Behavior modification techniques used to teach an animal to do something that is against its instincts or physical nature will probably be unsuccessful because of the _____.

24. Reinforcers—such as money, prizes, and praise—that are not inherently related to the activity being reinforced are called _____ reinforcers.

25. Sometimes called vicarious conditioning, _____ involves watching the behavior of another (a model) rather than experiencing that behavior directly.

26. The theories underlying _____ psychology have become increasingly influential, although strict behaviorists continue to reject them as vague and unnecessary.

behavior modification	extrinsic	punishment
biological constraints on learning	intermittent	reinforcer
cognitive	observational learning	token economy
extinction	operant	
	Pavlovian	

True-False

Read the following statements carefully and mark each true (T) or false (F).

27. ____ The dogs who salivated at the sound of a bell in the famous classical conditioning experiments learned to do so through the careful use of punishments and rewards.

28. ____ Classical conditioning may account for why some people seem to learn to be allergic to substances they have associated with ones to which they are already sensitive.

29. ____ Ivan Pavlov was the father of operant conditioning.

30. ____ The Skinner box was designed to catch rats for use in operant conditioning experiments.

31. ____ Responses learned through continuous reinforcement are the most resistant to extinction.

32. ____ Slot machines pay off (provide reinforcement) on a variable-ratio (VR) schedule.

33. ____ Punishment is perhaps the only certain method of behavior control.

34. ____ Behavior modification is employed almost entirely in experimental settings.

35. ____ The behavior modification system known as a token economy has proved particularly effective in institutional settings, such as prisons, mental hospitals, schools, factories, day-care centers, and nursing homes.

36. ____ The enjoyment of doing something and the satisfaction of accomplishment are intrinsic reinforcers.

37. ____ Behaviorists concentrate much of their attention on the role the human mind plays in shaping behavior.

Short-Answer Questions

As a final review exercise, write brief answers to demonstrate that you are achieving the learning objectives of this lesson.

1. Describe the process of classical (Pavlovian) conditioning and apply the principles in real-life situations.

2. Describe the process of operant conditioning and explain how the basic types of behavioral consequences affect learning.

3. Compare the effects of continuous reinforcement and intermittent schedules of reinforcement on learning.

4. Discuss several potential disadvantages of using punishment in real-world situations.

5. Define behavior modification and discuss its uses.

6. Explain how the modification of behavior can be complicated by such factors as the impact of intrinsic and extrinsic reinforcers and the biological constraints on learning.

7. Describe kinds of learning (e.g., latent learning and observational learning) that pose some problems for traditional conditioning theories and may require mentalistic explanations.

8. Distinguish between behavioral and cognitive explanations of behavior, and discuss why many psychologists consider both approaches when dealing with real-world problems.

Self-Test

1. Ivan Pavlov became the founder of classical conditioning as a result of
   a. his modifications of operant conditioning.
   b. research on digestion.
   c. studying children's fear of rats.
   d. training pigeons to play Ping-Pong.

2. The tendency, after conditioning, to respond to a stimulus that resembles one involved in the original conditioning is called
   a. extinction.
   b. spontaneous recovery.
   c. stimulus generalization.
   d. stimulus discrimination.

3. "Little Albert" was the 11-month-old subject of an experiment which included using conditioning to
   a. make him salivate when he heard a bell ring.
   b. cure him of his phobic (irrational) fear of rabbits.
   c. cure him of his phobic (irrational) fear of rats.
   d. establish a phobic (irrational) fear of rats in him.

4. Behavior, according to operant conditioning theories, is controlled by
   a. its consequences.
   b. free will.
   c. knowledge.
   d. instincts.

5. Which of the following reinforces behavior by removing something unpleasant?
   a. positive reinforcement
   b. negative reinforcement
   c. punishment
   d. extinction

6. Pavlov's favorite experimental subjects were dogs; Skinner is best known for using _____ as experimental subjects.
   a. monkeys and chimps
   b. white mice
   c. pigeons and rats
   d. children

7. In general, a reinforcer or punisher will have a greater effect
   a. if more than one person applies it.
   b. if its nature has been agreed upon by all concerned.
   c. the sooner it follows a response.
   d. the longer the intervals between its uses.

8. _____ produce extremely high, steady rates of responding, with responses quite resistant to extinction.

   a. Variable-ratio (VR) schedules of reinforcement

   b. Fixed-ratio (FR) schedules of reinforcement

   c. Fixed-interval (FI) schedules of reinforcement

   d. Continuous reinforcement

9. A basic principle of operant conditioning is that if you want a response to persist after it is learned, you should

   a. reinforce it continuously.

   b. reinforce it intermittently.

   c. not reinforce it.

   d. employ punishment when it is required.

10. Which of the following is NOT one of the serious disadvantages of using punishment to control behavior?

   a. It is often administered inappropriately.

   b. It tends to deprive the person being punished of attention.

   c. The recipient often responds with anxiety, fear, and rage, rather than improved behavior.

   d. Its effects may be temporary.

11. If the use of punishment is determined to be appropriate, it should

   a. always involve physical abuse.

   b. never be combined with positive reinforcement.

   c. be accompanied by information about what kind of behavior would have been more appropriate.

   d. be administered only by trained professionals.

12. Behavior modification is the application of conditioning techniques to reduce or eliminate _____ or _____ behavior or to teach new responses.

   a. reinforced; unreinforced

   b. positive; negative

   c. superstitious; phobic

   d. maladaptive; problematic

13. In a token economy, once a particular behavior is established, tokens can be phased out and replaced by more "natural" reinforcers, such as

    a. money.

    b. praise.

    c. rain checks.

    d. unconditioned stimuli.

14. Each of the following is a contention of critics of behaviorism **EXCEPT**

    a. They fear that its widespread use will crush creativity and turn people into sheep.

    b. They see operant conditioning as mechanistic, cold-blooded, and unethical.

    c. They object to the use of punishment or the withholding of reinforcers.

    d. They are certain society is too willing to use behavioral procedures to achieve inhumane goals.

15. Which of the following is **NOT** an extrinsic reinforcer?

    a. money

    b. prizes

    c. enjoyment of the task

    d. praise

16. In the modification of behavior, overdependence on extrinsic rewards can

    a. maximize the impact of punishment.

    b. undermine intrinsic motivation.

    c. cause instinctive drift.

    d. weaken stimulus control.

17. Grades received in school are _____ reinforcers that may do little to increase students' interest and motivation.

    a. extrinsic

    b. intrinsic

    c. primary

    d. natural

18. Latent learning occurs without obvious
    a. reason.
    b. preparation.
    c. reinforcement.
    d. assistance.

19. According to Albert Bandura, we also learn new responses by
    _____ the behavior of another.
    a. the overt response to
    b. classically conditioning
    c. observing
    d. shaping

20. In practice, behavioral and cognitive approaches are sometimes treated
    as
    a. utterly incompatible.
    b. in agreement on the basic causes of behavior.
    c. conflicting only because of the attitudes of individual practitioners.
    d. different levels of analysis, rather than as conflicting approaches.

21. For psychologists treating people in psychotherapy, to combine
    behavioral principles with cognitive ones is
    a. forbidden.
    b. unheard of.
    c. not unusual.
    d. standard practice.

Study Activities

The following activity challenges you to use your critical thinking and demonstrate how what you are learning can be applied to you and your own life. Try this activity and/or those your instructor assigns.

Psychological conditioning techniques are in use throughout modern society. Their employment is not confined to institutions, and the objects of their attention are not just troubled, disabled, or disturbed individuals. The purpose of this exercise is to begin discovering how pervasive the use of such techniques really is.

It would be impractical to do a telephone survey of therapists to ask them if they use methods based on classical and/or operant principles. Of course, you could contact professional organizations such as the American Psychological Association (APA) and inquire about the theoretical orientation of their members. But there is a far simpler way to get an indication of the degree to which psychological conditioning and behavior modification are relied upon by people in general and may even have become a part of western popular culture.

Go to your library and to several bookstores. List the titles of relatively new books (published within the last 10 or 20 years) on topics dealing with psychotherapy and mental health: problems in living, breaking habits, overcoming fears and phobias, compulsions and obsessions, shyness, addictive behavior, and all the other personal problems and psychological weaknesses to which each of us is prey. You will probably have a list of dozens of titles after your first stop. If you then look at several recent issues of *Publishers Weekly*, you should learn that many books of the sort you are investigating have been on the best-seller list. The fact that there is a market for such works is one sign of how much people have come to desire access to the methods of psychology—including, to a large degree, behavior modification techniques.

As you are compiling your list, be sure to read enough about the authors and the techniques discussed so you can determine what psychological approach each uses. Keep a tally of how many behaviorists, cognitive therapists, Gestalt psychologists, psychiatrists, and other practitioners you encounter. Then draw your conclusions, however tentative and less-than-authoritative they may be, about who is writing these books and about the many people who read them and who have confidence that psychology can give them aid and insight into the problems they encounter in everyday life.

Memory

Assignments

For the most systematic coverage of this lesson, we suggest that you complete the assignments in the sequence listed below.

Before viewing the video program:

- Read the "Learning Objectives" and "Overview" for this lesson. Use the Learning Objectives to guide your reading, viewing, and thinking.

- Read the "Viewing Notes" for this lesson.

- Read Chapter 10, "Memory," in the Wade and Tavris text. First, familiarize yourself with its contents by reading the Chapter Outline. As you read, note terms and concepts set in bold or italic type, especially those defined in the margins.

View the video program, "Memory"

After viewing the video program:

- Briefly note your answers to the questions at the end of the "Viewing Notes."

- Review all reading assignments for this lesson, including the Summary at the end of Chapter 10 in the textbook.

- Complete the "Review Exercises" to strengthen your understanding of this lesson's central concepts and terminology. Pay special attention to the "Vocabulary Check" exercise and the additional terms and concepts that follow—page references indicate where in the text assignment each term is defined. [Remember: there is a complete Glossary at the end of the text.]

- Take the "Self-Test" to measure the degree to which you are achieving this lesson's learning objectives. Check your answers against the "Answer Key" and review when necessary.

- Follow the suggestions in the "Study Activities" section at the end of this lesson and complete any other activities and projects assigned by your instructor.

Learning Objectives

When you have completed all assignments in this lesson, you should be able to:

1. Define memory.

2. Describe the three basic processes of memory: encoding, storage, and retrieval.

3. Describe the characteristics of the three memory systems in the so-called three-box model of memory: sensory memory, short-term memory, and long-term memory.

4. Explain the role of reconstruction in remembering information stored in long-term memory.

5. Describe three theories on why we forget long-term memories: interference, motivated forgetting, and cue-dependent forgetting.

6. Describe several mental strategies for improving memory.

7. Identify the major questions that scientists who study the biology of memory are trying to answer and describe at least one of the important lines of research they are pursuing.

8. Explain the importance of memory in daily life and to each individual's sense of identity.

Overview

You already know a great deal about memory. You know that some things are easier to remember than others: people and places associated with important moments in your life; great public events that moved you to experience fear, sadness, or elation; even the smallest piece of information that has been part of your life for many years. You are probably aware that not all information you are exposed to becomes part of your memories. Your rough ideas about memory and the fact that you may have a "good memory" have little to do with what memory really is and how it works.

This lesson introduces current theories or models of the nature of memory. It explains the **information-processing approach to memory** and identifies the basic processes involved in acquiring, retaining, and retrieving memories: **encoding**, **storage**, and **retrieval**.

The **sensory memory**, **short-term memory**, and **long-term memory** are described as the separate but interacting memory systems depicted by the **three-box model of memory**. Many examples and explanations clarify how each element operates, what distinguishes it from the others, and what role it plays in human experience.

People not only remember, they forget. An examination of theories about the process of forgetting—**decay**, **new memories replacing old**, **interference in memory**, **motivated forgetting**, and **cue-dependent forgetting**—reveals that forgetting is an important and provocative aspect of the study of memory.

This lesson includes useful and intriguing material on mental **strategies for improving memory** and on the serious matter of the untrustworthiness of **eyewitness testimony**.

Both the video lesson and the text illuminate exciting research on the **biological foundations of memory**. The video program includes straightforward explanations by some of the scientists who are beginning to reveal what goes on in the brain when it creates, retrieves, or loses memories. They explore the possible roles of **hormones** and **neurotransmitters** and of **neurons** and **synapses** in the memory process. Here you can learn about the long-range possibility of chemical enhancement or restoration of memory.

The importance of memory in daily life is self-evident, and this lesson explains why. It shows that your memory helps shape your self-identity. It examines such memory problems as **childhood amnesia** (why individuals have no recollection of their own lives from birth to age two or three). There is moving coverage in the video program of how a brain ailment such as **Alzheimer's disease** can rob people of memory and of the power to function normally.

The lesson makes it clear that all forms of memory, from fleeting sensory impressions to lifelong memories, are of central importance to your enjoyment of life and your capacity to function as a unique individual and a member of human society.

Viewing Notes

The video program "Memory" gives you direct access to some of the scientists whose research is revealing the nature and workings of memory. When you view this program, you will learn from the researchers themselves how they are uncovering the secrets of memory. You will hear them explain their theories and see the kind of laboratory work and clinical studies they and their colleagues are doing. You will witness what real people with memory disturbances experience and see what hope advances in memory research may offer to individuals with such impairments as amnesia and Alzheimer's disease.

As you watch the video program, consider the following questions:

1. What is it about events such as the *Challenger* space shuttle disaster and the assassination of President Kennedy that makes it possible for most people to remember in vivid detail what they were doing and how they felt at the time?

2. How does James McGaugh explain why laboratory animals' memory and ability to learn can be enhanced by biochemical agents?

3. How might McGaugh's research eventually be applied to human memory and learning, including impairments such as Alzheimer's disease?

4. How does Richard Granger employ computer models to simulate the memory processes that occur in living brains?

5. In what ways did the brain injury suffered by patient N. A. impair his memory?

6. What are some of the ways Alzheimer's disease disrupts the thinking of those it strikes?

7. Why does Curt Sandman think Alzheimer's disease involves more than biological and physical factors?

8. What concepts described in this video lesson have inspired therapeutic techniques that are proving to be successful in improving individuals' ability to learn and remember?

9. What does Elizabeth Loftus say about how the recollections of eyewitnesses can be distorted?

10. How do lawyers exploit the nature of the memory process to make the testimony of their witnesses more believable?

11. According to James McGaugh, what factors might make memory an undependable mechanism?

Review Exercises

Vocabulary Check

Match the following key terms and concepts with the appropriate definitions from the list below.

1. ___ childhood (infantile) amnesia (p. 380)

2. ___ chunk (p. 362)

3. ___ decay theory (pp. 376–377)

4. ___ encoding (p. 357)

5. ___ flashbulb memories (p. 351)

6. ___ maintenance rehearsal (p. 368)

7. ___ motivated forgetting (p. 378)

8. ___ neurotransmitters (video)

9. ___ proactive interference (p. 377)

10. ___ procedural memories (p. 364)

11. ___ rehearsal (p. 367)

12. ___ semantic memories (p. 365)

13. ___ sensory memory (pp. 358–359)

14. ___ source amnesia (p. 349)

15. ___ three-box model of memory (p. 359)

a. a theoretical model of memory describing three interacting memory systems: sensory memory, short-term memory, and long-term memory

b. repetition of information to improve retention and subsequent retrieval

c. vivid recollections of the details surrounding the perception of a significant or emotionally charged event

d. a meaningful unit of information; it may be composed of smaller units

e. forgetting recently learned material due to interference from information previously stored in memory

f.   the memory system that receives and momentarily holds information provided by the senses

g.   the theory that information (particularly in short-term memory) will eventually disappear if it is not reactivated

h.   rote repetition of material in order to maintain its availability in memory

i.   memories that reveal general knowledge such as facts, rules, concepts, and propositions

j.   memories required to carry out particular kinds of actions

k.   conversion of information into a form that can be stored in and later retrieved from memory

l.   the conscious or unconscious desire to eliminate painful or unpleasant experiences or information from memory

m.   the inability to distinguish what you originally experienced from what you heard or were told about an event later

n.   chemicals that carry messages between neurons

o.   a curious aspect of autobiographical memory: that most adults cannot recall any events from earlier than the third or fourth year of life

Other Key Terms and Concepts

Alzheimer's disease (video)

cognitive schema (p. 357)

computer models of memory process (video)

consolidation (p. 371)

cue-dependent forgetting (p. 378)

declarative (conscious) memories (p. 364)

deep processing (p. 368)

elaborative rehearsal (p. 368)

episodic memories (p. 365)

explicit memory (p. 355)

implicit memory (p. 357)

information-processing approach to memory (p. 357)

long-term memory (LTM) (pp. 358, 362)

long-term potentiation (p. 370)

memory (p. 348)

mnemonics (pp. 369, 385–386)

network models (p. 363)

parallel distributed processing models (PDP) (p. 359)

priming (p. 357)

recall (p. 355)

recognition (p. 355)

relearning method (p. 357)

retrieval (p. 357)

retroactive interference (p. 377; video)

serial-position effect (p. 365)

short-term memory (STM) (pp. 358, 361)

state-dependent memory (p. 378)

storage (p. 357)

synaptic change (video)

tip-of-the-tongue state (or phenomenon) (p. 363)

Completion

Fill each blank with the most appropriate term from the list of answers below.

16. The three basic memory processes are _____, _____, and _____.

17. The _____ is experienced when you are sure something is in long-term memory but you just can't recall it.

18. Memory appears to involve modifications in the _____, _____, and _____ of the neurons in the brain.

19. _____ devices are formal strategies, such as use of rhymes or formulas, for improving memory.

20. The memory process seems to involve neurotransmitters carrying chemical messages across the synapses between _____.

21. Memory is the capacity to _____ and _____ information and the structure or structures that make these processes possible.

22. Cognitive _____ refers to an integrated network of knowledge, beliefs, and expectations concerning a particular topic.

23. The _____ effect describes the tendency for items at the end of a list to be recalled readily.

24. The _____ model of memory describes the encoding, storage, and retrieval of information as operating through three separate but interacting memory systems: _____ memory, _____ memory, and _____ memory.

25. A significant or surprising event can produce _____ memories (vivid, detailed recollections of the event and the circumstances surrounding it).

26. The _____ school refers to therapists who believe that virtually all memories recovered in therapy should be accepted as true, whereas the _____ school comprises many research psychologists who argue that recovered memories are manufactured by therapists.

27. The behavior of tens of thousands of brain cells working in tandem can be simulated by _____ models of memory.

biochemistry	neurons	sensory
computer	recency	short-term
encoding	recovered-memory	storage
false-memory	retain (or store)	structure
flashbulb	retrieval	three-box
long-term	retrieve	tip-of-the-tongue state (or phenomenon)
mnemonic	schema	

True-False

Read the following statements carefully and mark each true (T) or false (F).

28. ____ The study of amnesia victims, such as Larry Squire's patient N. A., shows that the mechanisms of memory can be disrupted without necessarily causing other mental processes to deteriorate.

29. ____ The capacity of long-term memory is strictly limited, because as new memories are processed, they automatically replace older memories.

30. ___ Unless information in short-term memory is transferred to long-term memory, it is likely to decay and be lost forever.

31. ___ Amnesia always means the complete loss of existing memories and of the ability to acquire new memories.

32. ___ Eyewitnesses to crimes or accidents always have clear and unchanging images and concepts of what they experienced.

33. ___ Research has shown that true memories may be located in a different part of the brain from false memories.

34. ___ Because of the serial-position effect, it is harder to remember the items in the middle of a list than those at the beginning or the end.

35. ___ Experiences that trigger strong emotions are almost always easy to remember, so researchers can improve the memory and learning of laboratory animals by giving them hormones that artificially stimulate emotions usually experienced only during some exciting event.

36. ___ The fact that some very old long-term memories can be retrieved suggests that all memories from the past remain available.

37. ___ Computer models of the memory process are enabling researchers to begin to identify and understand the many interacting brain structures involved in memory.

Short-Answer Questions

As a final review exercise, write brief answers to demonstrate that you are achieving the learning objectives of this lesson.

1. Define memory.

2. Describe the three basic processes of memory: encoding, storage, and retrieval.

3. Describe the characteristics of the three memory systems in the so-called three-box model of memory: sensory memory, short-term memory, and long-term memory.

4. Explain the role of reconstruction in remembering information stored in long-term memory.

5. Describe three theories on why we forget long-term memories: interference, motivated forgetting, and cue-dependent forgetting.

6. Describe several mental strategies for improving memory.

7. Identify the major questions that scientists who study the biology of memory are trying to answer and describe at least one of the important lines of research they are pursuing.

8. Explain the importance of memory in daily life and to each individual's sense of identity.

Self-Test

1. From the biological perspective, memory is
   a. created by hormones.
   b. really very simple.
   c. changes in the nervous system produced by selective experience.
   d. mostly devoted to preserving unimportant events and experiences.

2. The information-processing approach defines memory as
   a. digital traces in the neurons of the cerebral cortex.
   b. the ability to think about one's experiences so the brain can store them in an organized fashion.
   c. conscious conversion of sensations into ideas.
   d. the capacity to retain and retrieve information.

3. Encoding is
   a. the modification of memories in response to stress.
   b. the conversion of information into a form the brain can process and store.
   c. a disruption of memory that prevents retrieval of information.
   d. the last stage of information processing necessary to store memories.

4. After encoding takes place, the next step in the processing of a memory is
   a. storage.
   b. retrieval.
   c. rehearsal.
   d. forgetting.

5. The model of memory involving sensory memory, short-term memory, and long-term memory is known as
   a. the pattern-recognition approach to memory.
   b. the computer model of memory.
   c. parallel distributed processing (PDP).
   d. the three-box model of memory.

6. The entry area of memory is

   a. sensory memory.

   b. short-term memory.

   c. long-term memory.

   d. the cerebellum.

7. David wants to be sure he remembers to take certain items to school. Before leaving the house, he repeats: "Lunch money, bus pass, latch key," several times. This is an example of

   a. elaborative rehearsal.

   b. maintenance rehearsal.

   c. deep processing.

   d. mnemonics.

In the blank next to each of the following definitions, write the letter of the most appropriate term or concept from the list that follows.

8. ___ maintenance rehearsal, elaborative rehearsal, and deep processing

9. ___ a network of knowledge, beliefs, and expectations concerning a particular topic

   a. cognitive schema

   b. retention strategies

10. Which of the following is **NOT** used to explain the organization of long-term memory?

   a. semantic memories

   b. sensory memories

   c. procedural memories

   d. episodic memories

11. Eyewitness testimony
    a.   can be depended upon if the event witnessed generated strong emotions in the witness.

    b.   requires eidetic imagery.

    c.   can be distorted by misinformation acquired long after the event witnessed and by the witness's honest efforts to reconstruct his or her memory of events.

    d.   can always be confirmed by use of a polygraph (lie detector).

12. The process whereby new information interferes with the ability to recall similar material already stored in memory is called
    a.   retroactive interference.

    b.   proactive interference.

    c.   retrograde amnesia.

    d.   encoding failure.

13. Motivated forgetting usually involves memories that are
    a.   associated with any strong emotion.

    b.   poorly encoded.

    c.   painful or unpleasant.

    d.   linked to many other memories.

14. Repeating a phone number over and over as a way of keeping it in short-term memory is called
    a.   retrieval.

    b.   rehearsal.

    c.   encoding.

    d.   forced recall.

15. Rhymes or formulas used to make it easier to remember something are called
    a.   chunks.

    b.   relearning methods.

    c.   elaborative rehearsal techniques.

    d.   mnemonic devices.

16. Most people's inability to describe the face of a penny accurately is due to their failure to employ which of the following techniques for improving memory?

    a. using visual imagery

    b. adding meaning

    c. paying sufficient attention

    d. encoding information in more than one way

17. Most scientists are convinced that the mechanisms of memory

    a. operate at the level of sensory organs.

    b. operate almost entirely automatically.

    c. involve chemical and structural changes at the level of neurons.

    d. are too complicated to be influenced by scientific efforts to improve individuals' ability to remember and to learn.

18. Which of the following is NOT one of the major lines of research being pursued by scientists studying the biology of memory?

    a. determining the roles of hormones and neurotransmitters

    b. gathering evidence that proves the ability to remember is inherited rather than learned

    c. discovering in what parts of the brain the mechanisms of memory operate

    d. using computers to model, measure, and test the memory process

19. The development of biochemical methods for improving human memory and treating such memory disorders as Alzheimer's disease

    a. has already been accomplished.

    b. is unlikely to be pursued, given the powerful negative side effects such substances are likely to have.

    c. might be possible within 20 years, in light of research such as James McGaugh's experiments using hormones to improve laboratory rats' ability to learn and remember.

    d. is acknowledged to be an impossible dream.

20. The principal explanation for childhood amnesia—the inability to remember personal experiences before age three or four—contends that it is due to

   a. repression resulting from some traumatic childhood event.

   b. the erroneous notion that events experienced by infants are important enough to remain in long-term memory.

   c. differences in styles of parenting and nurturing.

   d. the immaturity of the memory-processing structures of an infant's brain.

Read the following statements carefully and mark each true (T) or false (F).

21. ___ Alzheimer's disease may involve a patient's attitude and preferences as well as chemical/biological factors.

22. ___ Flashbulb memories involve only visual images.

23. ___ Events that stimulate your emotions are always easier to remember in detail.

Study Activities

These activities challenge you to use your critical thinking and demonstrate how what you are learning can be applied to you and your own life. Try those activities that interest you most and/or those your instructor assigns.

1. In Video Program 8, "Memory," the matter of eyewitness testimony is examined. An expert on the subject, Elizabeth Loftus, says that when a witness gets new information about an event—from other witnesses, the media, police, or attorneys—there is a potential for the new information, especially misleading information, to distort the witness's recollection.

   If you were a juror on a case such as that depicted in the courtroom scene in the video program, how would you evaluate the statements of the attorneys and the testimony of the witnesses and the defendant? Use what you have learned about how memory is received, stored, accessed, and altered to describe what kinds of remembered information are most likely to be reliable and what kinds are most likely to be untrustworthy. Identify the memory processes that cause these differences.

2. Can you memorize the following number and be able to recall it easily any time you want?

   557492201181828645904415661212560327712219163

   At first glance, any normal person would say memorizing such a long, seemingly random number would be all but impossible. But what if the number were not random and could be given meaning by breaking it into more manageable chunks? What if the first 9 digits were your own social security number? What if the next 11 were your telephone number? The next 6 might be the combination to a lock you use daily. Perhaps the next 11 are your best friend's telephone number, and maybe the final 7 digits indicate the date of your birth. After "chunking," the same set of digits would look like this:

   557-49-2201   1-818-286-4590   44-15-66   1-212-560-3277   12-2-1963

   That seemingly overwhelming long number is now a series of shorter numbers—chunks—that you can memorize and easily recall. In fact, you have already memorized such a number and many others much longer. Merely recalling all the telephone numbers you have already memorized would create a single, long number that might comprise dozens or even hundreds of digits.

   Think about this exercise and devise other variations of it. Use it as a reminder that you can improve your ability to remember by using mnemonic devices and practicing other memory-enhancing techniques.

Decision Making and Problem Solving

Assignments

For the most systematic coverage of this lesson, we suggest that you complete the assignments in the sequence listed below.

Before viewing the video program:

- Read the "Learning Objectives" and "Overview" for this lesson. Use the Learning Objectives to guide your reading, viewing, and thinking.

- Read the "Viewing Notes" for this lesson.

- Read Chapter 9, "Thinking and Intelligence," pages 305–324, 330–331, and 341, in the Wade and Tavris text. First, familiarize yourself with its contents by reading the Chapter Outline. As you read, note terms and concepts set in bold or italic type, especially those defined in the margins.

View the video program, "Decision Making and Problem Solving"

After viewing the video program:

- Briefly note your answers to the questions at the end of the "Viewing Notes."

- Review all reading assignments for this lesson, including the Summary at the end of Chapter 9 in the textbook.

- Complete the "Review Exercises" to strengthen your understanding of this lesson's central concepts and terminology. Pay special attention to the "Vocabulary Check" exercise and the additional terms and concepts that follow—page references indicate where in the text assignment each term is defined. [Remember: there is a complete Glossary at the end of the text.]

- Take the "Self-Test" to measure the degree to which you are achieving this lesson's learning objectives. Check your answers against the "Answer Key" and review when necessary.

• Follow the suggestions in the "Study Activities" section at the end of this lesson and complete any other activities and projects assigned by your instructor.

Learning Objectives

When you have completed all assignments in this lesson, you should be able to:

1. Explain the roles of concepts, propositions, and mental images in human reasoning.

2. Explain the roles and significance of subconscious and nonconscious mental processes.

3. Define reasoning and distinguish between inductive and deductive reasoning.

4. Define dialectical reasoning and explain its importance in solving real-world problems.

5. List and explain several sources of irrationality that can influence decision making.

6. List and describe the basic steps in the problem-solving process.

7. Distinguish between algorithms and heuristics as problem-solving strategies.

8. Explain how types of mental rigidity, such as mental set, can sometimes act as barriers to effective problem solving.

9. Discuss recent findings about creativity and contrast the roles of divergent and convergent thinking.

Overview

Even if you never studied this lesson, watched the video program, read the text assignment, or even took this course, you would still actively and regularly engage in decision making and problem solving. Even if you fail to acquire the information presented in this lesson, life in the real world will continue to demand that you weigh options and make decisions (good or bad), that you encounter problems and find (or fail to find) ways to solve them. What you learn here could help you improve the quality of your decision making and make you a more effective problem solver.

This lesson examines **thinking** and **reasoning**, introducing **concepts**, **propositions**, and **images** as elements of cognition, building blocks of thought that underlie reasoning. It explores the significance of **subconscious** and **nonconscious** mental processes. **Reasoning** is defined, and the sources of rationality and irrationality are identified. The differences between **inductive** and **deductive reasoning** are described. **Dialectical reasoning** is discussed in terms of its usefulness in confronting real-life problems that require the ability to think critically about opposing viewpoints.

The lesson identifies various aspects of **irrationality** that can influence decision making. The video program explains why illusions, biases, errors, and irrationality itself need not always be considered antithetical to effective decision making.

The lesson describes the information-processing strategies and the steps in the problem-solving process and explains such problem-solving approaches as **algorithms** and **heuristics**. Forms of mental rigidity, such as **mental set**, are shown to be pitfalls to problem solving.

The nature of **creativity** is examined, including the personality characteristics of creative individuals. Ideas on how to cultivate creativity and new ways to measure it are presented. Styles of creative thinking are discussed, and the differences between **convergent** and **divergent thinking** are highlighted.

Viewing Notes

The video program "Decision Making and Problem Solving" focuses on the idea that both rationality and irrationality influence human thought. It defines reasoning, explains the differences between decision making and problem solving, identifies the biases and other factors that limit our ability to make sound judgments, and describes the problem-solving process.

As you watch the video program, consider the following questions:

1. In the sixth-grade class's exercise on decision making, what do the students learn about identifying relevant facts and discounting biases that might affect good judgment?

2. How does Keith Holyoak distinguish deductive reasoning from inductive reasoning?

3. Why does Holyoak say that lots of important, everyday decision making requires the kind of skill we characterize as critical thinking?

4. According to Holyoak, what are some of the factors that can limit our ability to make sound judgments?

5. What are the essential differences between decision making and problem solving?

6. How does Robert Sternberg explain the problem-solving process?

7. What are some of the ways psychologists have found to help people, especially students, improve their reasoning skills and become better problem solvers?

8. What are psychologists learning about expert decision making and decision making under stress?

9. Is irrationality ever a positive factor in problem solving and decision making?

Review Exercises

Vocabulary Check

Match the following key terms and concepts with the appropriate definitions from the list below.

1. ____ algorithm (p. 310)

2. ____ concept (p. 306)

3. ____ convergent thinking (p. 341)

4. ____ creativity (p. 341)

5. ____ deductive reasoning (p. 310; video)

6. ____ dialectical reasoning (p. 312)

7. ____ divergent thinking (p. 341)

8. ____ heuristic (p. 312; video)

9. ____ inductive reasoning (p. 311; video)

10. ____ mental image (p. 307)

11. ____ mental set (p. 320)

12. ____ nonconscious processes (p. 308)

13. ____ reasoning (p. 310)

14. ____ thinking (p. 305)

a. a flexible, imaginative thought process leading to novel, but appropriate, solutions to problems, original ideas and insights, or new and useful products

b. a problem-solving strategy that is guaranteed to lead to a solution eventually

c. a tendency to solve a problem with the same strategies and rules used on previous problems

d. the drawing of conclusions or inferences from observations, facts, or assumptions

e. a mental representation that mirrors or resembles the thing it represents

f. a rule of thumb that guides problem solving but doesn't guarantee an optimal solution; often used as a shortcut in solving complex problems

g. reasoning in which the premises provide support for a certain conclusion, but the conclusion can still be false

h. mental processes occurring outside of and not available to conscious awareness

i.   a category that encompasses objects, relations, activities, abstractions, or quantities that have properties in common

j.   a process in which opposing facts or ideas are weighed and compared, for the purpose of determining the truth or resolving differences

k.   mental exploration of unusual or unconventional alternatives during problem solving, which tends to enhance creativity

l.   the mental manipulation of information stored in the form of concepts, images, or propositions

m.   reasoning in which a conclusion follows necessarily from certain premises; if the premises are true, the conclusion must be true

n.   thinking aimed at finding a single correct answer to a problem by applying knowledge and reasoning

Other Key Terms and Concepts

availability heuristic (p. 317)

basic concepts (p. 306)

cognitive dissonance (p. 321)

cognitive schema (p. 307)

confirmation bias (p. 318)

hindsight bias (p. 321)

irrationality (video)

justification of effort (p. 323)

metacognition (p. 330)

mindlessness (p. 308)

proposition (p. 306)

prototype (p. 306)

reflective judgment (p. 313)

subconscious processes (p. 308)

tacit knowledge (p. 331)

Completion

Fill each blank with the most appropriate term from the list of answers below.

15.   Football, baseball, basketball, and tennis are all instances of the _____ "sport."

16.   "Rocks are hard" and "psychology is hard" are _____.

17.   Mental processes that occur outside of conscious awareness but are accessible to consciousness when necessary are termed _____.

18.   If you start with one or more general assumptions, or premises, and draw a logical conclusion from them, you are employing _____ reasoning.

19. Because there is no one answer to many real-world problems, logic may have to be supplemented or replaced by _____ reasoning, a form of critical thinking in which opposing points of view are weighed and compared.

20. The role of _____ in decision making may be as great as or greater than that of facts or logic.

21. One contribution to irrationality in decision making is the _____, the tendency to overestimate the occurrence of an event because it is easily noticed, imagined, or remembered.

22. Among the basic information-processing strategies for problem solving are, in order: _____ the problem, _____ the problem, _____ a strategy, _____ the strategy, and _____ progress toward the goal.

23. In problem solving, the use of _____ is guaranteed to lead to a solution, whereas the use of _____ suggests a course of action but does not guarantee an optimal solution.

24. If you tend to try to solve new problems by using a strategy or procedure that worked on another problem, you are relying on a _____, which can be a barrier to problem solving.

25. Creative people tend to solve problems by employing _____ thinking, by considering unusual or unconventional alternatives, instead of relying solely on _____ thinking, which involves following a method or strategy that promises to lead to one correct solution.

26. Some personality characteristics often encountered in creative people are _____, _____, _____, _____, and _____.

algorithms	devising (selecting)	irrationality
availability heuristic	dialectical	mental set
concept	divergent	nonconformity
confidence	evaluating (or monitoring)	persistence
convergent		propositions
curiosity	executing (mastering)	recognizing (or identifying)
deductive	heuristics	
defining	independence	subconscious

True-False

Read the following statements carefully and mark each true (T) or false (F).

27. ____ Mental images can only occur as visual representations.

28. ____ Deductive reasoning often takes the form of a syllogism: a simple argument consisting of two premises and a conclusion.

29. ____ Juries arrive at their verdicts through use of deductive reasoning.

30. ____ One aspect of irrationality in decision making is the tendency to underestimate the probability of rare events.

31. ____ One of the basic steps in the problem-solving process must be defining the problem.

32. ____ Algorithms can be employed to solve almost any real-world problem.

33. ____ Mental sets make human learning and problem solving efficient and are particularly useful when a problem calls for fresh insights and methods.

34. ____ Critical thinking, or the use of reflective judgment, requires the ability to evaluate and integrate evidence, relate that evidence to a theory or opinion, and reach a conclusion that can be defended as reasonable or plausible.

35. ____ Highly creative people tend to prefer working alone.

36. ____ In general, creative people have narrow, tightly focused interests.

37. ____ A high IQ guarantees that you will be a creative individual.

Short-Answer Questions

As a final review exercise, write brief answers to demonstrate that you are achieving the learning objectives of this lesson.

1. Explain the roles of concepts, propositions, and mental images in human reasoning.

2. Explain the roles and significance of subconscious and nonconscious mental processes.

3. Define reasoning and distinguish between inductive and deductive reasoning.

4. Define dialectical reasoning and explain its importance in solving real-world problems.

5. List and explain several sources of irrationality that can influence decision making.

6. List and describe the basic steps in the problem-solving process.

7. Distinguish between algorithms and heuristics as problem-solving strategies.

8. Explain how types of mental rigidity, such as mental set, can sometimes act as barriers to effective problem solving.

9. Discuss recent findings about creativity and contrast the roles of divergent and convergent thinking.

Self-Test

1. A concept is a mental _____ that groups objects, relations, activities, abstractions, or qualities having common properties.

   a. image

   b. category

   c. exercise

   d. proposition

2. A mental representation of the relationships among concepts that expresses a unitary idea is called a(n)

   a. image.

   b. premise.

   c. proposition.

   d. prototype.

3. When you do something largely without thinking about each action you are performing, as when you drive a car while listening to the radio or talking on a cellular phone, your driving is a(n) _____ mental process.

   a. subconscious

   b. preconscious

   c. nonconscious

   d. unconscious

4. The mental processes that affect behavior but remain outside conscious awareness are

   a. subconscious.

   b. preconscious.

   c. nonconscious.

   d. unconscious.

5. Reasoning may best be thought of as a systematic method for drawing inferences or reaching conclusions from
    a. ideas, hypotheses, and theories.
    b. feelings, intuitions, and suspicions.
    c. concepts, images, and propositions.
    d. observations, facts, and assumptions.

6. Reasoning in which the premises provide support for the conclusion and may involve careful observations and the collection of evidence is called
    a. dialectical reasoning.
    b. deductive reasoning.
    c. inductive reasoning.
    d. a syllogism.

7. In deductive reasoning, the truth of the conclusion is
    a. guaranteed only if the premises upon which it is based are true.
    b. guaranteed regardless of the truth of the premises upon which it is based.
    c. guaranteed as long as at least one premise upon which it is based is true.
    d. not guaranteed.

8. Dialectical reasoning is most suitable for solving problems with
    a. undeniably true premises.
    b. only one answer.
    c. more than one "right" answer.
    d. no apparent answer at all.

9. Which of the following real-world situations would be LEAST suited to weighing and comparing opposing facts or ideas and resolving differences?
    a. a legislative debate over capital punishment
    b. drawing conclusions from facts gathered in a research project
    c. deliberations by a jury
    d. international arms control talks

10. Psychologists have shown that personal, economic, and political decisions cannot be explained without taking _____ into account.

    a. heuristics

    b. algorithms

    c. biases

    d. mindlessness

11. The tendency of people to overestimate the frequency and probability of catastrophic events that are widely and intensively reported in the media is called

    a. false expectation.

    b. the representativeness heuristic (or bias).

    c. the availability bias (or heuristic).

    d. relative accounting.

12. Which of the following would **NOT** be considered one of the basic steps in the problem-solving process?

    a. recognizing the problem

    b. denying there is a problem

    c. selecting a strategy

    d. carrying out the strategy

13. You can't begin to solve a problem until you have

    a. recognized the problem and defined exactly what it is.

    b. planned all the steps you will follow in problem solving.

    c. obtained professional advice and counseling.

    d. purged your mind of irrational conceptions.

14. It is important to monitor or evaluate each problem-solving strategy; if it isn't working or conditions affecting the problem change, then you should consider

    a. using a strategy that worked on some other problem.

    b. using a new strategy or repeating steps in the existing strategy.

    c. learning more about problem solving.

    d. giving up hope of overcoming that problem.

15. A problem-solving strategy that may consist of a set of rules or a recipe or could require trying all possible solutions is called a(n)

    a. heuristic.

    b. algorithm.

    c. syllogism.

    d. proposition.

16. A problem-solving technique that involves rules of thumb and trial-and-error and suggests a course of action rather than guaranteeing an optimal solution is called a(n)

    a. heuristic.

    b. algorithm.

    c. syllogism.

    d. proposition.

17. In complex real-world situations in which there is no obvious sequence of steps that will lead to a solution, _____ might prove most useful.

    a. inductive reasoning

    b. algorithms

    c. heuristics

    d. basic concepts

18. Developing a mental set can cause difficulty in problem solving because you may

    a. become too flexible and undisciplined in your thinking.

    b. have a tendency to try solving new problems using procedures that worked on previous problems.

    c. create a new set of procedures for each new problem.

    d. never have enough ideas in any one set.

19. Creative people

    a.   usually have very high IQs.

    b.   carefully follow a proven set of problem-solving steps.

    c.   work hard at a solution but know when to give up.

    d.   recognize that there may be more than one way to solve a
         problem.

20. Which of the following is **NOT** a personality characteristic found in
    most creative individuals?

    a.   curiosity

    b.   confidence

    c.   conformity

    d.   persistence

21. The video program contains a segment on creative problem solving
    under stress. The airline pilot who landed his plane even though it had
    a hole blown in its side and two failed engines

    a.   followed the rules in his manual without deviation.

    b.   relied on his experience and his ability to think fast and creatively
         in a novel and stressful situation.

    c.   was guided almost entirely by instructions from more
         knowledgeable experts on the ground.

    d.   was lucky in that he had been through a similar crisis before and
         knew just what to do this time.

22. Which of the following is most likely to motivate creative activity?

    a.   the desire for money

    b.   an opportunity to get attention

    c.   the wish to avoid punishment

    d.   a sense of accomplishment

Study Activities

The following activity challenges you to use your critical thinking and demonstrate how what you are learning can be applied to you and your own life. Try this activity and/or those your instructor assigns.

Decision making and problem solving can be highly theoretical or extremely practical. A mathematician may spend a lifetime trying to solve a problem that has defied solution for generations. An inventor such as Thomas Edison may try hundreds of possible ideas or materials before finding the one that makes a new device work as it should. Such problem solving remains beyond the experience and understanding of most of us, but all of us must make decisions and solve problems every day, and our problem-solving abilities can influence the quality of our lives. Your ability to make correct decisions and solve problems can improve your chances of being happy and successful in your personal and professional life. Bad decision making and problem solving can fill your life with frustration and failure—and can even endanger your life.

The following exercise provides many opportunities to test your decision-making and problem-solving skills on supremely practical matters ranging from personal comfort to survival itself.

Consider what you might have to do if your community was struck by a major earthquake, hurricane, or other disastrous event. Think of all the problems you might have to solve and all the unavoidable decisions you could be called upon to make. Would you be sufficiently creative to solve problems despite the lack of resources and outside assistance? Would you have planned ahead to improve your chances of dealing with such an emergency?

For example, if an earthquake trapped you inside your home, how would you get out? Do you know what exits are available to you? Are there escape routes you haven't thought of before? If you had to dig or pry or bash your way out, what tools would you use? If you had no real tools (or were denied access to them by the quake), how would you fashion makeshift tools?

If an earthquake or hurricane drove you from your home without any money or identification, what are some of the first things you'd do to normalize your life? Do you have any idea how you'd prove who you are? How would you go about obtaining new identification; whom would you get to verify your identity; who might be able to provide you with shelter, food, money? Whether you will have to turn to others—friends and family, charitable organizations, the government—or can rely on yourself will depend largely on your having planned ahead of time to deal with a disaster and on your energy and creativity in handling novel problems that are sure to arise during an emergency.

Again, if you were confined to your home, how would you solve some of the most basic problems presented by major emergencies? If power lines were cut, what would you do for light and heat, or for cooking? If you hadn't stocked batteries for flashlights, would you have candles, a way to make a fire? What might you use to make a cooking fire in? Do you know, or can you figure out, ways to get light or make a fire when the switches are all dead and there may not even be any matches? Similarly, how would you get water? Without an emergency supply, how would you obtain water to drink and to use for cooking and bathing? Though it is an unpleasant problem to contemplate, with water lines out, could you devise a practical and reasonably hygienic way to dispose of human bodily waste?

Plan in detail, in writing, what you would need and how you would act in an emergency. You should create a scenario of what might happen in a disaster that leaves you on your own for three or four days. Write down all the problems you might have to solve—including very specific descriptions of what you think you would have to do. Be realistic about what can occur, but be imaginative about how you might cope with real problems. If you share your home with others, you may want to solicit their ideas as well. Yet remember that most creative thinking is a solitary act.

Clearly, this is not a frivolous exercise, not a game. Disasters happen all too frequently, catching people unprepared and unable to find ways to solve the problems that threaten to overwhelm them. You may never have to cope with a natural disaster, but preparing a survival strategy and amassing emergency rations and materials ahead of time should be common sense. It doesn't take a disaster to test your capacity to solve problems. On any day, anywhere, you could lock yourself out of your car, be faced with an emergency repair job that calls for a tool or fastener you just don't have, or need to help someone who is injured (or help yourself). You could give up and call for help, or you could practice divergent thinking: use your belt for a tourniquet; use a pair of panty hose to stop a radiator hose from leaking; sacrifice a cassette tape to hold a bandage firmly in place. The possibilities are endless: the possible problems you might be called upon to solve and the possible answers that a mind open to innovative solutions might find.

Review the lesson material on problem solving and creativity, paying particular attention to the "Taking Psychology with You" section on becoming more creative (page 341 in the Wade and Tavris textbook). Keep in mind that it doesn't matter if a problem is monumental or minute, historic or ordinary. It's an important problem if it's *your* problem.

Lesson 10

Language

Assignments

For the most systematic coverage of this lesson, we suggest that you complete the assignments in the sequence listed below.

Before viewing the video program:

- Read the "Learning Objectives" and "Overview" for this lesson. Use the Learning Objectives to guide your reading, viewing, and thinking.

- Read the "Viewing Notes" for this lesson.

- Read Chapter 3, "Evolution, Genes, and Behavior," pages 72–76; Chapter 9, "Thinking and Intelligence," pages 336–340; and Chapter 14, "Development over the Life Span," pages 504–505, in the Wade and Tavris text. First, familiarize yourself with their contents by reading the Chapter Outlines. As you read, note terms and concepts set in bold or italic type, especially those defined in the margins.

View the video program, "Language"

After viewing the video program:

- Briefly note your answers to the questions at the end of the "Viewing Notes."

- Review all reading assignments for this lesson, including the Summaries at the end of Chapters 3, 9, and 14 in the textbook.

- Complete the "Review Exercises" to strengthen your understanding of this lesson's central concepts and terminology. Pay special attention to the "Vocabulary Check" exercise and the additional terms and concepts that follow—page references indicate where in the text assignment each term is defined. [Remember: there is a complete Glossary at the end of the text.]

- Take the "Self-Test" to measure the degree to which you are achieving this lesson's learning objectives. Check your answers against the "Answer Key" and review when necessary.

- Follow the suggestions in the "Study Activities" section at the end of this lesson and complete any other activities and projects assigned by your instructor.

Learning Objectives

When you have completed all assignments in this lesson, you should be able to:

1. Define what is meant by language and describe its important characteristics.

2. Evaluate the debate over research into whether or not animals can acquire language skills.

3. Summarize the debate on the influence of language on thought, including Whorf's theory.

4. List and describe the basic stages of language development in children.

5. Discuss the interrelationship between biological readiness and social interaction in language development, and describe some of the ways parents and other caregivers help children learn speech.

Overview

Obviously, if you are reading these words you are able to use language. You no doubt acquired language skills as a small child. Unless you've actually studied the subject, you, like most people, probably haven't thought about what a remarkable capability language is. As the video program for this lesson puts it: "Language is perhaps the highest achievement of human cognition."

This lesson defines **language** and explains what makes **meaningfulness**, **displacement**, and **productivity** essential characteristics of language. **Grammar** and **syntax** are described. The distinction between the **surface structure** and **deep structure** of sentences is explained.

The intriguing, often touching, and always controversial subject of animals' ability to acquire and use language is dealt with in the text assignment and in the video lesson.

The lesson addresses the debate over the degree to which language influences thought and thought influences language. Benjamin Lee Whorf's **linguistic relativity theory** (which holds that language molds habits of thought and perception and that different language communities therefore tend to have different views of reality) is examined. Research in this field is discussed in the video lesson.

Both the text and the video program describe children's acquisition of language, discussing and demonstrating the basic stages in children's development of language skills, from cooing and **babbling**, through **telegraphic speech** and one-word sentences, to the ability to use and understand complex sentences and the rules of grammar.

The lesson deals with the issue of whether language is somehow innate or is acquired almost entirely through learning and social interaction. Noam Chomsky's concept of a **language acquisition device** (of children being biologically ready to use language because human brains are prewired that way) is introduced. Considerable evidence is offered to show that children's development of language skills depends heavily on their interaction with parents and other caregivers.

The video program also has an interesting segment on how specific parts of the brain produce and comprehend language. It focuses on language disorders that can be caused by damage to those areas of the brain.

Viewing Notes

The video program for this lesson characterizes language as the basis for all human social interaction. It explains that language is a product of learning and environmental influences but is also part of the human genetic endowment, saying that our brains appear to be biologically programmed to enable us to learn, use, and understand language. The program identifies the essential characteristics of language, evaluates the research into whether or not animals can acquire language skills, details the stages of language development in children, and discusses factors which influence that development. The program shows how scientists have learned much about the nature of humans' ability to use and comprehend language by studying language disorders caused by damage to parts of the brain that facilitate speech and language.

As you watch the video program, consider the following questions:

1. According to Patricia Greenfield, what are the three important, if not essential, characteristics of human language?

2. How have methods developed to teach chimpanzees to use symbols to communicate been employed to help retarded children?

3. Is Harold Chipman's statement that babies are "born communicators," and that their acquisition of language depends on their interaction with others and with their environment, at all contradictory?

4. How does Chipman characterize the stages through which children pass in developing language skills?

5. What does Patricia Zukow mean when she says that the interaction between caregivers and children acquiring language helps the children crack the linguistic code?

6. How does Susan Curtiss explain what it means "to have a grammar"?

7. What do Chipman and Curtiss say about the human capacity for language being innate, part of the human genetic endowment?

8. What does Eran Zaidel say about how language is organized in the brain and about language disorders caused by damage to the brain?

9. What did Greenfield discover from her experiment with Zinacantecan children about the influence of language on thought?

Review Exercises

Vocabulary Check

Match the following key terms and concepts with the appropriate definitions from the list below.

1. ___ anthropocentrism (p. 340)

2. ___ aphasia (video)

3. ___ deep structure (p. 73)

4. ___ displacement (p. 337; video)

5. ___ grammar (p. 73; video)

6. ___ language (pp. 73, 337–338)

7. ___ language acquisition device (p. 73)

8. ___ linguistic relativity theory (Whorfian hypothesis) (video)

9. ___ overregulation (video)

10. ___ parentese (baby talk) (p. 504; video)

11. ___ signs (p. 72)

12. ___ syntax (pp. 73, 506)

13. ___ telegraphic speech (p. 505; video)

a. the set of grammatical rules governing the way words may be arranged to form sentences and convey meaning

b. the notion that language shapes thought and perception and that speakers of different languages have different views of reality

c. a child's first combinations of words, which omit nonessential words

d. the tendency to falsely attribute human qualities to nonhuman beings

e. the ability to combine elements that are themselves meaningless into an infinite number of utterances that convey meaning

f. the tendency of young children to grasp a grammatical rule and then overgeneralize it

g. the system of linguistic rules governing sounds (or gestures, in the case of sign languages), meanings, and syntax of a language; may be viewed as the mechanism for generating all possible sentences in a language

h. an innate mental module, according to Noam Chomsky, that allows young children to develop language if they are exposed to an adequate conversation sample

i. the capacity of language to permit communication about objects and events that are not present here and now

j. a disorder of language due to some form of brain damage after language has normally been acquired

k. gestural signals that, like sounds do, convey both abstract and concrete ideas; from their form you usually can't guess their meaning

l. a stylized type of speech adults around the world tend to use when speaking to young children

m. the underlying meaning of a sentence

Other Key Terms and Concepts

anthropomorphism (p. 340)

babbling phase (p. 504)

cognitive ethology (p. 337)

critical period (for language acquisition) (p. 76)

meaningfulness (p. 337; video)

overregularization (p. 74)

productivity (p. 337; video)

psycholinguistics (p. 73)

surface structure (p. 73)

universal grammar (p. 74)

Completion

Fill each blank with the most appropriate term from the list of answers below.

14. The essential characteristics that make a communication system qualify as a language are _____, _____, and _____.

15. You can use your knowledge of syntax to figure out how the _____ of a sentence as it is actually spoken or written reveals an underlying _____ that contains its meaning.

16. The rules of _____ tell us which strings of sounds and words (or, in sign language, which gestures) form acceptable utterances in a given language and which do not.

17. One of the factors that cast doubt on some studies of the ability of apes to acquire language skills was the discovery that researchers may have been unwittingly prompting the animals' behavior with _____.

18. The fact that people in different cultures have various ways of describing the same phenomena—as, for example, the Inuit having many different words for snow—provided Benjamin Whorf evidence with which to develop his _____, which holds that individuals' native language powerfully influences their _____ and _____.

19. Cognitive ethology is the study of cognitive processes in _____.

20. All infants go through a _____ between the ages of about 6 months and 1 year.

21 "More candy," "here Mommy," and "allgone juice" are examples of the so-called _____ used by children just beginning to use combinations of words to communicate.

22. Language acquisition seems to depend on both _____ and _____.

23. Parents and other caregivers in many cultures help children learn speech by speaking to them in _____, a slower, simpler, repetitious form of adult language.

24. There may be a critical period, during the first 5 to 10 years of life, when children's language development depends most on _____ and _____.

babbling phase	meaningfulness	productivity
biological readiness	nonhuman animals	social experience (interaction)
close human relationships	nonverbal cues	surface structure
deep structure	parentese (baby talk)	telegraphic speech
displacement	perception	theory of linguistic relativity
grammar	practice in conversation	thought

True-False

Read the following statements carefully and mark each true (T) or false (F).

25. ___ Language refers solely to meaningful spoken communication.

26. ___ The difference between "You need a new car" and "A new car needs you" is a matter of syntax.

27. ___ The surface structure of a sentence carries its actual meaning.

28. ___ Research on the ability of apes to acquire language skills has been totally discredited, and such studies are no longer conducted.

29. ___ There is evidence suggesting that in each culture the language may influence the acquisition of specific mental skills by guiding attention in particular directions.

30. ___ The theory of linguistic relativity, which holds that language determines thought, has remained unchallenged since it was conceived by Benjamin Whorf.

31. ___ Children demonstrate the ability to produce two- and three-word combinations of words long before they develop a repertoire of symbolic gestures.

32. ___ The ease of learning language is much greater in the young child than in the older child or the adult.

33. ___ Noam Chomsky is best known for developing new methods to teach children language skills.

34. ___ Some experts assert that children's acquisition of language depends not so much on learning but on the human brain's biological programming to acquire language and the rules of grammar.

35. ___ A child's language is not creative or original, but comes merely from imitating or passively parroting adults.

Short-Answer Questions

As a final review exercise, write brief answers to demonstrate that you are achieving the learning objectives of this lesson.

1. Define what is meant by language and describe its important characteristics.

2. Evaluate the debate over research into whether or not animals can acquire language skills.

3. Summarize the debate on the influence of language on thought, including Whorf's theory.

4. List and describe the basic stages of language development in children.

5. Discuss the interrelationship between biological readiness and social interaction in language development, and describe some of the ways parents and other caregivers help children learn speech.

Self-Test

1. The main purpose of language is to make _____ reference to things, ideas, and feelings.
    a. symbolic
    b. specific
    c. meaningful
    d. truthful

2. The ability of language to allow the expression and comprehension of an infinite number of novel utterances, created on the spot, is known as
    a. meaningfulness.
    b. displacement.
    c. productivity.
    d. fluency.

3. _____ is the part of grammar that governs how words are arranged to convey meaning.
    a. Linguistics
    b. Syntax
    c. Surface structure
    d. Deep structure

4. What a written or spoken sentence says, regardless of its underlying meaning, is called its
    a. surface structure.
    b. deep structure.
    c. grammar.
    d. syntax.

5. _____ communicate.
    a. Only humans
    b. Only humans, chimpanzees, and gorillas
    c. Only animals that possess language skills
    d. Virtually all animals

6. In the efforts to teach apes to communicate with sign language and similar communication systems, which of the following was **NOT** a problem detected by skeptics and by some researchers themselves?

   a. Researchers were unwittingly giving the animals nonverbal cues.

   b. Researchers were unable to achieve sufficient rapport with these lower animals to maintain interest in teaching them language skills.

   c. The animals appeared to be stringing signs and symbols together haphazardly merely to earn rewards.

   d. Researchers may have been insufficiently objective; in their optimism and their affection for the animals, they sometimes overinterpreted the animals' behavior.

7. The latest studies into whether or not animals can acquire language skills have

   a. failed to overcome the methodological weaknesses identified in earlier studies.

   b. improved because researchers have switched their attention from chimps and gorillas to dolphins and whales.

   c. benefited from the criticism of earlier research methods and are a marked improvement over past research.

   d. not shown that they have any application to human communication problems.

8. The notion that language shapes thought is usually associated with

   a. Noam Chomsky.

   b. George Orwell.

   c. B. F. Skinner.

   d. Benjamin Lee Whorf.

9. Cultural evidence, such as the fact that the Hopi language has no past, present, or future tenses, helped support the

   a. concept of linguistic universals.

   b. theory of linguistic relativity.

   c. education of native Americans.

   d. rules of grammar.

10. Which of the following best describes the position that most experts would now take in the debate over the relationship between language and thought?

    a. Language controls thought.

    b. A person who speaks one language can only experience reality in one way.

    c. All the languages of the world are basically alike.

    d. Language appears to influence thought in some ways, but thought also influences language.

11. Which of the following is **NOT** characteristic of most children in the initial stages of developing language skills?

    a. babbling

    b. telegraphic speech

    c. knowledge of the rules of grammar

    d. one-word sentences

12. Which of the following accounts for the fact that children everywhere seem to go through similar stages of linguistic development?

    a. All languages have the same basic structure.

    b. Children are born with a sort of "universal grammar."

    c. All parents use the same techniques to prompt their children to develop language skills.

    d. The United Nations has been successful in promoting international uniformity in language training and development.

13. Deprivation studies of children whose language development was delayed or impaired point to the fact that

    a. the basic stages of language development can be initiated at almost any age.

    b. if a critical stage of language development is missed, the deprivation may never be overcome.

    c. impairment in early language development can easily be remedied later, in school.

    d. language does not develop in stages that build on one another.

14. The language acquisition device is

    a. Benjamin Lee Whorf's concept of why people who speak different languages experience reality in different ways.

    b. Noam Chomsky's idea of an innate mental module that allows children to develop language if they are exposed to an adequate conversation sample.

    c. B. F. Skinner's notion of how children learn language through operant conditioning.

    d. computerized instructional hardware and software developed to aid students learning new languages.

15. Rewarding children for saying the right words and punishing them for making errors

    a. usually has little effect on their acquisition of language.

    b. is the best way to help them learn language skills.

    c. only works with highly motivated children.

    d. is what makes the language acquisition device work.

16. Children's language development seems to depend

    a. largely on the knowledge and instructional skills of their parents or other caregivers.

    b. entirely on their genetic endowment.

    c. entirely on social interaction.

    d. both on biological readiness and social experience.

17. Which of the following kinds of behavior by parents or other caregivers is LEAST likely to facilitate children learning how to talk and to increase their language skills?

    a. using books, games, flash cards, or computer learning devices to drill an infant or toddler in grammar rules

    b. speaking in a simplified form of adult language

    c. repeating and modifying something a child has said incorrectly, thereby providing a model of correct speech

    d. repeating exactly, and even amplifying, a child's correct utterances

Study Activities

The following activity challenges you to use your critical thinking and demonstrate how what you are learning can be applied to you and your own life. Try this activity and/or those your instructor assigns.

One segment of the video program deals with language disorders caused by damage to the brain. Such disorders, generally known as **aphasia**, help researchers understand the roles different brain structures play in making it possible for human beings to acquire, comprehend, and use language. (You may want to review pages 120–123 in Chapter 4 of the Wade and Tavris text for background on the localization of function in the cerebral cortex.) As a study activity, you might try to learn more about this subject. You should be able to sharpen your research skills while improving your knowledge of language disorders and of the brain.

You could start by building a basic bibliography. At the library, consult the subject index for books and articles on language and the brain, on hemispheric specialization, on the temporal lobes (where language function is localized), and on Broca's area and Wernicke's area of the brain. Your bibliography should include selections you have read and books or articles by authors prominently mentioned in other writings. From the reading materials you examine, you will be able to acquire detailed information on how particular parts of the brain are involved in speech and language. You should also obtain a clear and complete definition of aphasia. For this, you might want to look at dictionaries and encyclopedias devoted to psychological, psychiatric, and biomedical subjects.

As you gather data on this subject, preserve and organize it. You might want to start a file or notebook. It could contain your bibliographical entries; notes on your reading; the names of significant researchers and clinicians and descriptions of their experiments, discoveries or treatments; definitions of key terms and concepts; and pictures, drawings, or any other written or graphic material that illustrates your topic.

See where this research project leads you. How far you go, how detailed you make your project, depends on how much the subject captures your interest and how intrigued you become with the search for information and understanding. You can also speak with your instructor about the possibility of getting extra credit in the course for this research itself and/or for a report that might be produced from it.

Lesson 11

Emotion

Assignments

For the most systematic coverage of this lesson, we suggest that you complete the assignments in the sequence listed below.

Before viewing the video program:

- Read the "Learning Objectives" and "Overview" for this lesson. Use the Learning Objectives to guide your reading, viewing, and thinking.

- Read the "Viewing Notes" for this lesson.

- Read Chapter 11, "Emotion," in the Wade and Tavris text. First, familiarize yourself with its contents by reading the Chapter Outline. As you read, note terms and concepts set in bold or italic type, especially those defined in the margins.

View the video program, "Emotion"

After viewing the video program:

- Briefly note your answers to the questions at the end of the "Viewing Notes."

- Review all reading assignments for this lesson, including the Summary at the end of Chapter 11 in the textbook.

- Complete the "Review Exercises" to strengthen your understanding of this lesson's central concepts and terminology. Pay special attention to the "Vocabulary Check" exercise and the additional terms and concepts that follow—page references indicate where in the text assignment each term is defined. [Remember: there is a complete Glossary at the end of the text.]

- Take the "Self-Test" to measure the degree to which you are achieving this lesson's learning objectives. Check your answers against the "Answer Key" and review when necessary.

- Follow the suggestions in the "Study Activities" section at the end of this lesson and complete any other activities and projects assigned by your instructor.

Learning Objectives

When you have completed all assignments in this lesson, you should be able to:

1. List the three basic elements that are apparently factors in all emotions and explain the concepts that are helping to resolve the historic conflict over the roles and relative importance of mind and body in human emotion.

2. Discuss the special relationship between emotions and facial expressions.

3. Describe the effects of epinephrine and norepinephrine on arousal and emotions, explain why these hormones alone cannot produce emotions, and discuss methods of managing anger.

4. Summarize research findings associating emotions with specific brain regions.

5. Describe the varieties of emotion and discuss how culture influences the experience and expression of emotion.

6. Identify several ways in which emotions are communicated.

7. Discuss the importance of gender to the experience and expression of emotions.

Overview

If an infant sticks its tongue out at you, you probably smile or laugh. If an adult you're arguing with does the same thing, you surely get angrier. The difference in response is because the baby's behavior communicates something far different from the identical facial expression of an adult. This lesson explores **emotions** and their communication, a subject that is fundamental to human psychological and social experience. Included is an intriguing analysis of the differences between such seemingly similar emotions as envy and jealousy and shame and guilt.

In this lesson, the body, mind, and culture are identified as playing a role in all emotions. Physiological, cognitive, and cultural factors are discussed in detail. The lesson addresses the long-standing debate over whether emotion is more a matter of body or of mind and introduces some findings and research that are helping to resolve this historic conflict.

The fascinating subject of the facial expression of emotions is covered at some length in both the text and the video program, including definition of **facial feedback**. The discussion identifies universal facial expressions but also explains that their recognition can depend on the social context in which they are seen.

The process of **arousal**, including the role of the adrenal hormones **epinephrine** and **norepinephrine**, is explained. The text and video cover the special importance of **anger** and its management. There is discussion of the scientific evidence associating emotions with specific regions of the brain.

There is revealing coverage of how an individual's mental state can influence emotions. Schachter and Singer's **two-factor theory of emotion** is explained. As an example of the interaction of thoughts and feelings, the problem of depression is closely examined.

The lesson deals with the variety of emotions and their expression. There is intriguing information on the influence of culture on how, when, where, and whether emotions should be expressed (**display rules**) and on whether emotion must be communicated in response to social and cultural expectations even when it is not actually felt (**emotion work**). The ways emotions are communicated, including such nonverbal means as **body language**, are examined.

Differences in the ways men and women express and experience emotions are discussed, with reference to biological and cultural forces that impinge on each of us.

Viewing Notes

This video program explains and illustrates the universality of certain human emotions. The important findings of Paul Ekman and his colleagues are discussed in some detail by Ekman himself. He describes his fascinating work on how facial expressions communicate various emotions and traces the various directions his research has taken over the years. Another video segment focuses on anger, how it is expressed, and how it may be managed. Textbook author Carol Tavris, whose research includes the study of anger, appears in this video program to contrast some traditional notions about how to deal with anger with what she believes are more effective measures based on a more accurate understanding of what anger really is and can do. In the final part of the program, the relationship between performance and emotion is dramatically portrayed. Commentary by sports psychologist Michael Mahoney and Frank Leyden, former head coach of the Utah Jazz basketball team, is combined with action footage of basketball star Karl Malone to demonstrate the impact (positive and negative) of emotion on performance.

As you watch the video program, consider the following questions:

1. What are emotions and how do we experience them?

2. What emotions seem to be most basic, most commonly communicated through facial expressions by people all over the world?

3. Why did Paul Ekman have to extend his research on facial expression beyond the developed world to places such as New Guinea?

4. What does Ekman say about the interaction of biological and cultural forces on the communication of emotion?

5. What is Ekman's Facial Action Coding System (FACS)?

6. What is the relationship between anger and aggressive behavior, as discussed by Raymond Novaco?

7. How does Carol Tavris's analysis of anger run counter to some commonly held beliefs about how anger should be regarded and handled?

8. What are some of Tavris's strategies for managing anger?

9. How does the video segment on basketball star Karl Malone explain the relationship between emotion and performance anxiety?

Review Exercises

Vocabulary Check

Match the following key terms and concepts with the appropriate definitions from the list below.

1. ___ amygdala (pp. 397–398)
2. ___ arousal (p. 398)
3. ___ body language (pp. 410–411)
4. ___ display rules (p. 409; video)
5. ___ emotion (p. 392; video)
6. ___ emotion work (pp. 411, 415)
7. ___ epinephrine, norepinephrine (adrenaline, noradrenaline) (p. 398)

8. ___ Facial Action Coding System (FACS) (video)
9. ___ facial feedback (p. 395)
10. ___ primary emotions (p. 406)
11. ___ secondary emotions (p. 406)
12. ___ two-factor theory of emotion (p. 401)

a. expression of an emotion in response to role requirements rather than because of what a person really feels

b. the method that allows researchers to analyze and identify each facial muscle and combination of muscles that are associated with various emotions

c. a state involving a pattern of facial and bodily changes, cognitive appraisals, subjective feelings, and tendencies toward action—the experience and expression of which are shaped by culture

d. the theory that emotions depend on both physiological arousal and a cognitive interpretation or evaluation of that arousal

e. the level of energy that allows the body to respond quickly

f. a small structure in the limbic system that appears to be responsible for evaluating sensory information and quickly determining its emotional importance

g. adrenal hormones that provide fuel and feeling for all emotional states

h. countless nonverbal signals of body movement, posture, gesture, and gaze

i. emotions that are either "blends" of emotions or that are specific to certain cultures

j. the process by which the facial muscles send messages to the brain, identifying the emotion a person feels

k. emotions that are considered universal and biologically based

l. social and cultural rules that regulate when, how, and where a person may express (or suppress) emotional feelings

Other Key Terms and Concepts

anger (pp. 396, 406; video)

attributions (pp. 402–403)

cognitive interpretation
(pp. 401–402)

neurocultural theory (p. 393)

physiological arousal
(pp. 401–402)

Completion

Fill each blank with the most appropriate term from the list of answers below.

13. The basic elements, in addition to arousal, that apparently are factors in all emotions are the _____, the _____, and the _____.

14. In the process of _____, the facial muscles send messages to the brain, identifying emotions that a person feels.

15. When you face some demanding environmental situation, the sympathetic nervous system instructs the adrenal glands to release _____ and _____, which produce a state of _____—a level of energy that allows your body to respond quickly.

16. In their efforts to identify parts of the brain responsible for different aspects of the emotional experience, researchers have traced elements of universal emotions such as fear, rage and sexual desire to the _____ system and the _____.

17. According to the _____ theory of emotion proposed by Stanley Schachter and Jerome Singer, emotion depends on _____ and the _____ of that arousal.

18. _____ are the explanations that people make to account for their own and other people's behavior.

19. All cultures recognize positive (pleasant) and negative (unpleasant) emotions; researchers have further distinguished _____ emotions, which appear to be universal, and _____ emotions, which include cultural variations and blends or degrees of emotion.

20. Every society has _____ that regulate how and when emotions may be expressed.

21. Men and women differ in how, when, and where they _____ some emotions.

22. Men are more likely than women to express anger, fear, and hurt pride in the form of _____.

aggressive action	display rules	mind
arousal	epinephrine	norepinephrine
attributions	express	physiological
body	facial feedback	arousal
cognitive interpretation	hypothalamus	primary
	limbic	secondary
culture		two-factor

True-False

Read the following statements carefully and mark each true (T) or false (F).

23. ____ Research on emotion has moved us a long way toward resolving the historic conflict between the mind ("reason") and the body ("emotion"). Rather than regarding reason and emotion as separate, often conflicting processes, researchers now emphasize the ways in which physiological and cognitive processes interact.

24. ____ Human emotions depend on a complex combination of physiological responses and mental processes.

25. ____ Human emotions involve the mind and the body, and people's emotions are seldom influenced by their culture.

26. ____ People all over the world use very similar facial expressions to communicate certain basic emotions.

27. ____ In stressful situations, your sympathetic nervous system releases epinephrine and norepinephrine into your bloodstream to prevent you from becoming too aroused.

28. ___ Many psychologists agree that it is usually best to express anger rather than hold it in.

29. ___ People are likely to experience more than one emotion at a time.

30. ___ Depression is a purely physiological phenomenon independent of the depressed person's cognitions.

31. ___ Fear and anger are universal primary emotions found among human beings in every known society.

32. ___ Only women have to hide the emotions they feel and pretend to experience emotions they don't feel.

33. ___ There is considerable evidence that women feel emotions more often and more intensely than men do.

Short-Answer Questions

As a final review exercise, write brief answers to demonstrate that you are achieving the learning objectives of this lesson.

1. List the three basic elements that are apparently factors in all emotions and explain the concepts that are helping to resolve the historic conflict over the roles and relative importance of mind and body in human emotion.

2. Discuss the special relationship between emotions and facial expressions.

3. Describe the effects of epinephrine and norepinephrine on arousal and emotion, explain why these hormones alone cannot produce emotions, and discuss methods of managing anger.

4. Summarize research findings associating emotions with specific brain regions.

5. Describe the varieties of emotion and discuss how culture influences the experience and expression of emotion.

6. Identify several ways in which emotions are communicated.

7. Discuss the importance of gender to the experience and expression of emotions.

Self-Test

1. Which of the following is **NOT** one of the three basic elements that seem to be factors in all emotions?
    a. physiological changes in the body and face
    b. genetic programming of psychological reactions
    c. cognitive processes, such as interpretations of events
    d. cultural influences that shape the experience and expression of emotion

2. Regarding emotions, the interaction between mind and body
    a. starts with the body and the mind responds.
    b. starts with the mind and the body responds.
    c. works in both directions.
    d. starts with the culture and influences the body and mind at the same time.

3. Emotions, cognitions, and their interconnections
    a. remain largely the same from right after birth.
    b. evolve and change in the course of an individual's development.
    c. only manifest themselves when an individual is old enough to respond to cultural influence.
    d. are little affected by anything but physiological processes.

4. The research of Paul Ekman, Wallace Friesen, and other modern psychologists indicates that
    a. the expression of primary emotions varies greatly from one society to another.
    b. the basic, universal facial expressions do not necessarily communicate the primary emotions.
    c. few human beings can control their facial expressions to mask their emotions.
    d. all human beings express primary emotions in much the same way: as an innate tendency, not as a result of learning.

5. The purpose of universal facial expressions is probably to
   a. help each individual develop an identifiable appearance.
   b. communicate with others.
   c. release pent-up emotions.
   d. cover genuine emotions.

6. Ekman and his associates developed a special coding system that
   a. identifies the differences in facial expressions between members of different societies.
   b. identifies the basic facial expressions that communicate the primary emotions.
   c. analyzes the dozens of facial muscles to see how they are associated with various emotions.
   d. reveals psychological problems requiring professional psychological intervention.

7. Epinephrine (with or without norepinephrine)
   a. only produces physiological arousal associated with fear and anger.
   b. is only involved in powerful emotional states, such as rage.
   c. provides the feeling of an emotion: the tingle, excitement, and sense of energy.
   d. is no longer considered to play a significant role in the mechanism of arousal and emotion.

8. Which of the following is NOT one of the reasons why it takes more than just epinephrine and norepinephrine to produce emotions?
   a. Arousal takes several forms and may involve different parts of the brain and different hormones.
   b. Some people experience arousal and emotions even though their adrenal glands are no longer able to produce epinephrine and norepinephrine.
   c. The concept of arousal doesn't distinguish one emotion from another or emotions in general from other states of excitement.
   d. Two individuals may have different emotional responses to the same situation.

9. According to research by Carol Tavris and others, managing your anger by letting it out, by freely expressing it, is

    a. likely to prolong it and make you feel worse.

    b. better than keeping it bottled up.

    c. the best way to respond to other people's anger.

    d. unlikely to have much impact on you or those toward whom you direct your anger.

10. Research to identify specific areas of the brain that may be responsible for emotions has determined that

    a. the left cerebral hemisphere is responsible for anger and fear and the right hemisphere for joy.

    b. the limbic system (especially the amygdala) and hypothalamus are involved with universal emotions and their regulation.

    c. "pleasure centers" and "rage circuits" are found throughout the brain.

    d. emotion is controlled by environmental and cultural forces, not the brain.

11. Contemporary research on the role of the brain in emotion

    a. focuses on discovering particular structures of systems, such as rage circuits or pleasure centers.

    b. hopes to locate the brain's emotion center so that its surgical removal or control by chemicals can free people of emotion and make them wholly rational.

    c. emphasizes the interactions between emotion and cognition in different parts of the brain.

    d. is proving that emotion is a vestige of human beings' animal origins and is controlled entirely by the more "primitive" parts of the brain.

12. Because emotions must be recognized, identified, interpreted, analyzed, and responded to, the "thinking" part of the brain, the _____, must play a role in emotions.

    a. limbic system

    b. cerebral hemispheres

    c. hypothalamus

    d. reticular activating system (RAS)

13. Two people participated in the same successful enterprise, but one remembers feeling uplifted and joyful at the outcome and the other recalls being depressed and miserable. Which of the following probably best explains these differences in emotion?

    a. There were variations in each person's production of epinephrine and norepinephrine.

    b. The people's parents had come from different societies.

    c. Different regions of each person's brain reacted to the experience.

    d. The two people thought about and explained the experience differently.

14. Which of the following would NOT be used to characterize secondary emotions?

    a. They include cultural variations.

    b. They are universal and biologically based.

    c. They may be blends of different feelings.

    d. They may involve degrees of emotional intensity.

15. Experts generally agree that the primary emotions include

    a. fear, anger, and joy.

    b. disgust, anger, and shame.

    c. love, joy, and sadness.

    d. fear, anger, and hatred.

16. Acting out an emotion you don't really feel, but which is expected of you by your culture or social situation, is called

    a. a secondary emotion.

    b. arousal.

    c. emotional range.

    d. emotion work.

17. Every society has _____ that govern how and when emotions may be expressed.

    a. contractual agreements

    b. display rules

    c. ethnic imperatives

    d. body language

18. Nonverbal (and even unconscious) communication through posture, gestures, body movements, and gaze is called

    a. emotion work.

    b. display rules.

    c. body language.

    d. body English.

19. Body language seems to be _____ in the communication of emotion.

    a. imperative

    b. important

    c. unimportant

    d. rare

20. Which of the following is **NOT** true?

    a. Women are more likely than men to express negative emotions, such as fear and embarrassment, to close friends and family.

    b. Men usually express emotions such as fear to their male friends.

    c. Men are more likely than women to display negative feelings aggressively.

    d. Within any given cultural group, neither sex experiences normal, everyday emotions more than the other.

21. Women in the United States tend to smile more than men do, because

    a. their social and economic situation makes them so happy.

    b. they experience so much that is funny and entertaining.

    c. it helps them to pacify, nurture, and convey deference as part of their emotion work.

    d. men, by comparison, are grumpy and unhappy.

Study Activities

These activities challenge you to use your critical thinking and demonstrate how what you are learning can be applied to you and your own life. Choose those activities that interest you most and/or those your instructor assigns.

1. Collect faces. Because the face is where emotion is most visible, it is worthwhile to improve your ability to identify various emotions reflected by facial expressions. Review pages 393–396 in the Wade and Tavris textbook and recall the segments in the video in which Paul Ekman explains his research on how people all over the world communicate basic emotions through certain universal facial expressions. You may also want to consult some of Ekman's writings, several of which are listed in the textbook's bibliography.

   You can do informal research by collecting pictures of facial expressions from magazines and newspapers. Choose facial expressions that most clearly indicate particular emotional states—from basic ones such as fear, surprise, and anger to more subtle ones like contempt and shame. You might want to take your own photographs, but don't instruct your subjects to make faces. Use candid shots that capture genuine emotions. Continue this project until you've collected several examples of as many emotions as possible and are confident that you can discern the differences in facial expression that communicate differences in emotion.

2. Compile a dictionary of gestures. This exercise can be fun as well as enlightening. After reviewing pages 408–410 in the Wade and Tavris textbook, create a gesture dictionary from your observations of the people around you, from the mass media, even from your own behavior and your memories. Write down your observations, describing what you see or recall and defining what you think each gesture means. For example, if you're driving and someone gestures at you, carefully describe the physical character of the gesture and whether it was a friendly wave, a threatening signal, or something else. Watch the ways people use their heads, arms, hands, fingers, or entire body posture to communicate emotion. You may wish to collect pictures to go with your descriptions and definitions. Continue the project as long as you continue encountering new gestures.

3. Chart your own emotions. Review pages 403–405 in the Wade and Tavris textbook and examine the variety, range, and complexity of your own emotional reactions. Ask yourself how you respond to various experiences, how emotional you get, and what forms your emotions take. If you continue this exercise for several weeks, you should begin to detect patterns—wide swings, ups and downs, or emotional responses that tend to cluster within a narrow range.

Lesson 12

Motivation

Assignments

For the most systematic coverage of this lesson, we suggest that you complete the assignments in the sequence listed below.

Before viewing the video program:

- Read the "Learning Objectives" and "Overview" for this lesson. Use the Learning Objectives to guide your reading, viewing, and thinking.

- Read the "Viewing Notes" for this lesson.

- Read Chapter 12, "Motivation," pages 421–422, 441–452; Chapter 13, "Theories of Personality," pages 467–470, 472–475; Chapter 3, "Evolution, Genes, and Behavior," pages 70–71, 84–89; Chapter 9, "Thinking and Intelligence," pages 321–323, 341; and Chapter 8, "Behavior in Social and Cultural Context," pages 272–274, in the Wade and Tavris text. First, familiarize yourself with their contents by reading the Chapter Outlines. As you read, note terms and concepts set in bold or italic type, especially those defined in the margins. Take the Quick Quizzes to check your understanding of material being described and explained.

View the video program, "Motivation"

After viewing the video program:

- Briefly note your answers to the questions at the end of the "Viewing Notes."

- Review all reading assignments for this lesson, including the Summaries at the end of Chapters 12, 13, 3, 9, and 8 in the textbook.

- Complete the "Review Exercises" to strengthen your understanding of this lesson's central concepts and terminology. Pay special attention to the "Vocabulary Check" exercise and the additional terms and concepts that follow—page references indicate where in the text assignment each term is defined. [Remember: there is a complete Glossary at the end of the text.]

- Take the "Self-Test" to measure the degree to which you are achieving this lesson's learning objectives. Check your answers against the "Answer Key" and review when necessary.

- Follow the suggestions in the "Study Activities" section at the end of this lesson and complete any other activities and projects assigned by your instructor.

Learning Objectives

When you have completed all assignments in this lesson, you should be able to:

1. Define motivation and indicate its relationship to the study of emotions.

2. List and briefly describe the basic kinds of motivational conflict.

3. Describe the basic principles of drive theory and discuss its limitations for explaining many human actions.

4. Explain the set-point theory of weight control.

5. Discuss curiosity and play as behavioral motives.

6. Explore the role of consistency (consonance) as a cognitive motive and explain cognitive dissonance theory.

7. Discuss the importance of attachment and affiliation as deep emotional needs.

8. Explain how the following factors can affect achievement motivation: expectations and values, need for competence, need for achievement, culture, gender, and need for power.

9. Identify key intrinsic and extrinsic motivating factors that can influence how a person performs in the work, school, or personal environment.

10. Describe Abraham Maslow's hierarchy of needs theory and explain several problems with this theory.

Overview

This lesson investigates **motivation**: what makes human beings do what they do. It examines the drives that push us and the incentives that pull us toward some goal. It comments on the relationship between motivation and emotion and lists the kinds of motivational conflicts people typically encounter: **approach-approach**, **approach-avoidance**, **avoidance-avoidance**, and **multiple approach-avoidance**.

The basic principles of **drive theory** are explained, and the role of drives in human motivation is contrasted to that of social **motives**. An intriguing concept, the **set-point theory** of weight control, is discussed in some detail.

The lesson examines **curiosity** and **play** as behavioral motives, considering how people (and some animals) are motivated by both **novelty** and **familiarity**. It also explores people's need for consistency and understanding and explains why **cognitive dissonance** is sufficiently unpleasant that people make strenuous efforts to liquidate it and bring their thoughts, feelings, and behaviors back into balance.

A large part of the lesson is devoted to **social motives** and factors that can affect motivation. **Attachment** and **affiliation** are identified as deep emotional needs. The **need for competence**, the **need for achievement**, and the **need for power** are shown to be basic, yet complex, motives for why some people perform, succeed, and excel. The motivational role of expectations and values is explained, and **self-fulfilling prophecies** are discussed. The degree to which gender and culture increase or reduce **achievement motivation** is also considered.

The video program introduces and defines **extrinsic** and **intrinsic motivations**. It explains how their interplay can influence one's performance in school, at work, and in other settings. The section "The Effects of Work on Motivation" (pages 444–446 in the Wade and Tavris textbook) examines factors in the workplace that can improve workers' motivation, satisfaction, achievement, and effectiveness.

A discussion of Abraham Maslow's famous **hierarchy of needs theory** identifies ways in which it still seems a valid approach to understanding motivation and pinpoints aspects of the theory that have been called into question.

Viewing Notes

The video program provides dramatic examples of what motivates people. It amplifies the text's explanation of why people think, behave, and make choices as they do. Several experts clarify why motivation is such a complex process, involving biological, sociocultural, and personality factors. The program deals with some spectacular extremes in behavior. It examines why people are motivated to entertain themselves through thrill seeking or to take high-risk jobs. The program pays particular attention to what motivates individuals at work and in school, identifying what makes them choose one job over another and what makes them try to perform, succeed, and excel.

As you watch the video program, consider the following questions:

1. How important is the correlation between motivation and performance, and between motivation and achievement?

2. To what extent does motivation depend on individual differences?

3. What are some of the biological, sociocultural, and personality factors that contribute to human motivation?

4. Why do individuals engage in thrill seeking and take dangerous jobs like performing stunts for the movies?

5. Why is the interplay between intrinsic and extrinsic motivations so important, especially in work and school settings?

6. What does attribution theorist Bernard Weiner say about the role of expectancy and self-esteem in human motivation?

7. Why are teachers—especially those who give their students opportunities to make choices—crucial in determining children's motivation to study and learn?

8. Why does behavioral psychology (reinforcement theory) play a relatively minor role in explaining motivation, whereas attribution theory and other aspects of cognitive psychology seem central to understanding motivation?

9. How important are emotions and such concepts as love, fun, and play to human motivation?

10. What makes perceptions so important to motivation?

11. What aspects of Maslow's hierarchy of needs theory seem to be considered valid, and what aspects are subjects of controversy?

Review Exercises

Vocabulary Check

Match the following key terms and concepts with the appropriate definitions from the list below.

1. ___ attribution theory (p. 272; video)

2. ___ cognitive dissonance (p. 321)

3. ___ extrinsic motivation (p. 341; video)

4. ___ "glass ceiling" (p. 446)

5. ___ hierarchy of needs (p. 450; video)

6. ___ intrinsic motivation (pp. 341, 452; video)

7. ___ monochronic (p. 474)

8. ___ motivation (pp. 421–422; video)

9. ___ need for achievement (nAch; achievement motivation) (p. 442)

10. ___ need for affiliation (p. 424; video)

11. ___ need for power (p. 443)

12. ___ self-efficacy (p. 467)

13. ___ self-fulfilling prophecy (p. 468)

14. ___ set point (p. 84)

15. ___ social motives (video)

a. a state of tension that occurs when a person simultaneously holds two cognitions that are psychologically inconsistent or when a person's belief is inconsistent with his or her behavior

b. the motive to associate with other people, as by seeking friends, moral support, contact comfort, or companionship

c. according to one theory, a homeostatic mechanism that regulates food intake, fat reserves, and metabolism to keep an organism at its predetermined weight

d. Abraham Maslow's idea that human motives range from simple biological needs to complex psychological ones, and that the lower needs must be met before higher ones can be addressed

e. the tendency to act on expectations in such a way as to make them come true

f. a process within a person or animal that causes that organism to move toward a goal

g. learned motives, such as the need for affiliation, power, and competence

h. a learned motive to meet personal standards of success and excellence in a chosen area

i. a person's belief that he or she is capable of producing desired results

j. term that describes people or cultures that organize time into linear segments

k. a learned motive to dominate, influence, or control others

l. a barrier to promotion that is so subtle as to be transparent, yet strong enough to prevent advancement

m. motivation based on external incentives, such as pay, praise, attention, or the avoidance of punishment

n. the theory that people are motivated to explain their own and others' behavior by attributing causes of that behavior to a situation or a disposition.

o. motivation based on internal rewards, such as the basic pleasure of the activity itself, the intellectual challenge, or the satisfaction of curiosity

Other Key Terms and Concepts

attachment (p. 422)

drive theory (p. 421; video)

expectations (p. 441; video)

mastery (learning) goals (p. 448)

motivational conflicts (pp. 449–450; video)

performance goals (p. 448)

polychronic (p. 474)

values (p. 441; video)

Completion

Fill each blank with the most appropriate term from the list of answers below.

16. Both _____ and _____ come from the Latin root meaning "to move."

17. When you are equally attracted by two or more possible activities or goals, you may experience a(n) _____ motivational conflict; when one activity or goal has both a positive and a negative aspect, a(n) _____ motivational conflict may occur.

18. According to _____, biological needs result from states of physical deprivation, which, in turn, produce a physiological drive, a state of tension that motivates a person (or animal) to satisfy the need.

19. Your _____ body weight is the weight you stay at when you aren't thinking about it, when you aren't trying to gain or lose; it is the weight you tend to return to after you've made efforts to get above or below it.

20. When reality doesn't match expectations, _____ is the motive that impels us to find reasons for such contradictions.

21. Leon Festinger's theory of _____ predicts how people will receive and process information that conflicts with their existing ideas.

22. Human infants (in fact, all young primates) seem to become attached to their mothers, or other caretakers, for the _____ adults provide, because being touched, held, and cuddled is as important to them as receiving food.

23. Your expectations can create a _____ because of your tendency to behave in a way that will make the prediction come true.

24. Competence requires more than ability; it seems to involve a belief in _____, the conviction that you can successfully accomplish what you set out to do.

25. Your motivation for work might include such extrinsic (external) factors as _____ and _____ and such intrinsic (internal) factors as _____ and _____.

26. One problem with Abraham Maslow's hierarchy of needs was its apparent failure to account for people being motivated to address several needs _____, even if those needs were on more than one level of Maslow's hierarchy.

approach-approach	emotion	self-efficacy
approach-avoidance	fame	self-fulfilling prophecy
cognitive dissonance	happiness	set-point
contact comfort	intellectual satisfaction	simultaneously
curiosity	money	
drive theory	motivation	

True-False

Read the following statements carefully and mark each true (T) or false (F).

27. ___ Physical needs play a much greater role in human motivation than social motives (learned motives) do.

28. ___ Motivation and emotion are often studied together. Although both processes involve cognition as well as physiology, they are not synonymous; emotion is only one kind of motivating force.

29. ___ In approach-avoidance motivational conflicts you must choose between "the lesser of two evils."

30. ___ Avoidance-avoidance motivational conflicts require you to choose between "the lesser of two evils."

31. ___ The set-point theory of weight control has yet to be supported by human or animal research.

32. ___ Human beings have deep affection for the familiar and also have great curiosity about the new, novel, or unknown.

33. ___ According to the theory of cognitive dissonance, the harder you work to achieve a goal, the more you will value it, even if, objectively, the goal turns out to be less desirable than it appeared to be when you began working toward it.

34. ___ Of all the social motives, the need for affiliation is the only one most people can get along without.

35. ___ In modern western societies, not only are there differences in the distribution of power between men and women, but research also shows that women do not even seem to have a need for power.

36. ___ In the workplace, "merit pay" for special achievement can enhance not only extrinsic motivation but also intrinsic motivation, because it rewards people for doing good work, not merely for showing up for work.

37. ___ The idea of a hierarchy of needs and motives is popular, especially with business managers, because Maslow's original theory has been verified by scientific research.

Short-Answer Questions

As a final review exercise, write brief answers to demonstrate that you are achieving the learning objectives of this lesson.

1. Define motivation and indicate its relationship to the study of emotions.

2. List and briefly describe the basic kinds of motivational conflict.

3. Describe the basic principles of drive theory and discuss its limitations for explaining many human actions.

4. Explain the set-point theory of weight control.

5. Discuss curiosity and play as behavioral motives.

6. Explore the role of consistency (consonance) as a cognitive motive and explain cognitive dissonance theory.

7. Discuss the importance of attachment and affiliation as deep emotional needs.

8. Explain how the following factors can affect achievement motivation: expectations and values, need for competence, need for achievement, culture, gender, and need for power.

9. Identify key intrinsic and extrinsic motivating factors that can influence how a person performs in the work, school, or personal environment.

10. Describe Abraham Maslow's hierarchy of needs theory and explain several problems with this theory.

Self-Test

1. Motivation is defined as a process within a person (or animal) that causes that organism to move toward
   a. a goal or away from an unpleasant situation.
   b. all other organisms.
   c. a homeostatic state.
   d. higher levels in the hierarchy of needs.

2. Emotion
   a. means the same thing as motivation.
   b. is one kind of motivating force.
   c. will only motivate a person who doesn't have strong social goals.
   d. involves physiology alone, whereas motivation involves only cognition.

3. In _____ motivational conflicts, one goal or activity both attracts and repels you.
   a. approach-approach
   b. approach-avoidance
   c. avoidance-avoidance
   d. multiple approach-avoidance

4. In _____ motivational conflicts, you must choose between "the lesser of two evils."
   a. approach-approach
   b. approach-avoidance
   c. avoidance-avoidance
   d. multiple approach-avoidance

5. A series of studies on how students dealt with motivational conflicts revealed that

   a. only approach-approach conflicts seemed insoluble.

   b. only avoidance-avoidance conflicts seemed insoluble.

   c. most conflicts will resolve themselves if ignored.

   d. the failure to resolve conflicts can cause physical and mental distress.

6. According to drive theory, biological needs result from states of physical _____, which, in turn, produce a physiological _____, a state of tension that motivates a person (or animal) to satisfy the need.

   a. excitement; change

   b. change; need

   c. deprivation; drive

   d. deprivation; need

7. Drive theory cannot account for all human motivation because

   a. biological needs are so easily satisfied.

   b. not everyone has biological drives strong enough to motivate them.

   c. people also have social motives, which are as important as biological needs.

   d. the homeostatic mechanism operates only in cold climates.

8. Set-point theory holds that

   a. being overweight is a symptom of psychological problems.

   b. being overweight is caused by overeating.

   c. once a person reaches his or her set-point body weight, neither dieting nor overeating will be able to change it.

   d. an interaction of metabolism, fat cells, and hormones works to keep each person's body at a predetermined weight.

9. According to set-point theory, _____, _____, and _____ are regulated by a complex set of physiological mechanisms.

   a. food intake; fat reserves; metabolism

   b. metabolism; fat cells; hormones

   c. culture; ethnic background; heredity

   d. needs; drives; attitudes

10. _____ novelty seems to be a part of the human evolutionary heritage.

   a. An intolerance for

   b. An acceptance of

   c. An attraction to

   d. A fear of

11. _____ engage in so-called practice play, behavior that prepares them for serious adult activities.

   a. Only the young of predators, such as cats,

   b. Only human children

   c. Only human children who are pressured to do so by their parents or caregivers

   d. The young of many species

12. The state of tension that occurs when a person simultaneously holds two cognitions (thoughts, beliefs) that are psychologically inconsistent, or holds a belief that is incongruent with his or her behavior, is called

   a. cognitive balance.

   b. cognitive dissonance.

   c. homeostasis.

   d. extrinsic motivation.

13. One of the most popular methods of reducing dissonance is
    a. shifting responsibility.

    b. denying the importance of the decision.

    c. justification of effort.

    d. assuming that everyone else would make the same decision.

14. Studies of close relationships find that
    a. both sexes suffer when a love relationship ends if they did not want it to.

    b. women depend on men more than men depend on women.

    c. men depend on men more than women depend on women.

    d. because most men tend to fear closeness, few men form lasting intimate attachments.

15. Albert Bandura argues that _____ involves a belief in self-efficacy, the conviction that you can successfully accomplish what you set out to do.
    a. achievement

    b. competence

    c. power

    d. affiliation

16. Research has shown that whether people facing difficult problems experience a sense of mastery or helplessness is unrelated to their ability and seems to depend more on whether they are motivated by _____ or _____.
    a. biological needs; social needs

    b. emotions; beliefs

    c. mastery (learning) goals; performance goals

    d. attraction; repulsion

17. Intrinsic motivators are generated by
    a. the task itself.

    b. the need for something in addition to extrinsic rewards.

    c. what one's family, friends, or boss says.

    d. a natural resistance to outside pressure, even when it is positive.

18. Which of the following is an intrinsic motivation to do well in school?
    a. getting good grades

    b. pleasing your family

    c. the chance to make more money

    d. the joy of learning

19. According to Abraham Maslow, human beings behave badly—in ways that diminish their humanness—only when
    a. they fail to achieve self-actualization.

    b. they achieve higher goals, such as self-actualization, but fail to meet lower needs.

    c. their lower needs are frustrated, especially their needs for love, belonging, and self-esteem.

    d. they have very few biological needs and many psychological ones.

20. After analyzing some of the problems with Maslow's theory, it might be safest to say that
    a. biological needs always take precedence over psychological needs.

    b. human beings are incapable of being motivated by such elevated needs as self-actualization and self-transcendence.

    c. Maslow did prove that human needs must always be organized vertically, so that each requires fulfillment before the next can be met.

    d. each of us develops an individual hierarchy of motives during development from childhood to old age.

Study Activities

These activities challenge you to use your critical thinking and demonstrate how what you are learning can be applied to you and your own life. Try those activities that interest you most and/or those your instructor assigns.

1. Based on this lesson, determine if you have had, or are now having, motivational conflicts, and evaluate your method of handling them.

   Like most people, you have probably been attracted to two or more activities or goals and have had to choose between them. It may have been something as simple as being in the mood for pizza and for burgers at the same time. It could have been as serious as believing you were in love with two different people. Such approach-approach conflicts can be troublesome, but they are usually more pleasant than avoidance-avoidance conflicts, in which you must choose between two undesirable alternatives.

   Honestly think about your past and present experiences with motivational conflicts. Write down what kinds of conflicts you've confronted, and ask yourself how you resolved each. It is all right to get used to this exercise by describing almost any motivational conflict. However, as you start to figure out what is really being asked of you, try to concentrate on relatively important conflicts—things like deciding whether to go to college or start a career or deciding on one job offer over another. Indicate how you felt when you realized you faced such conflicts and while you were trying to resolve them.

   The goal of this activity is not to prove whether or not you are good at resolving motivational conflicts. The idea is to make you aware that such conflicts are natural and normal aspects of life. You should be ready to try to deal with how they make you feel and to meet the demands they place upon you.

2. Ask yourself what factors play the greatest role in motivating you to perform in school, at work, and in your personal life. Provide written answers to the following questions and others that may emerge as you think about this subject. Do you consider yourself driven to demonstrate competence, to achieve, or to attain power? In the goals you pursue, do you find that your gender increases or decreases your motivation and your chances for success? Do you respond more to extrinsic motivators, such as money and fame, or to intrinsic ones, such as the sheer love of doing something? What are your goals, where are you heading, what do you want to accomplish, and what sort of person do you want to be?

Be thorough and candid in your self-analysis. Make an effort to see yourself as others see you and to identify your goals and the kinds of motivational fuel that drive you toward them.

Gender and Relationships

Assignments

For the most systematic coverage of this lesson, we suggest that you complete the assignments in the sequence listed below.

Before viewing the video program:

- Read the "Learning Objectives" and "Overview" for this lesson. Use the Learning Objectives to guide your reading, viewing, and thinking.

- Read the "Viewing Notes" for this lesson.

- Read Chapter 12, "Motivation," pages 422–423, 426–440; Chapter 14, "Development over the Life Span," pages 513–517; and Chapter 3, "Evolution, Genes, and Behavior," pages 65, 77–80, in the Wade and Tavris text. First, familiarize yourself with their contents by reading the Chapter Outlines. As you read, note terms and concepts set in bold or italic type, especially those defined in the margins. Take the Quick Quizzes to check your understanding of material being described and explained.

View the video program, "Gender and Relationships"

After viewing the video program:

- Briefly note your answers to the questions at the end of the "Viewing Notes."

- Review all reading assignments for this lesson, including the Summaries at the end of Chapters 12, 14, and 3 in the textbook.

- Complete the "Review Exercises" to strengthen your understanding of this lesson's central concepts and terminology. Pay special attention to the "Vocabulary Check" exercise and the additional terms and concepts that follow—page references indicate where in the text assignment each term is defined. [Remember: there is a complete Glossary at the end of the text.]

- Take the "Self-Test" to measure the degree to which you are achieving this lesson's learning objectives. Check your answers against the "Answer Key" and review when necessary.

- Follow the suggestions in the "Study Activities" section at the end of this lesson and complete any other activities and projects assigned by your instructor.

Learning Objectives

When you have completed all assignments in this lesson, you should be able to:

1. Explain why psychologists disagree over whether sex should be considered a primary drive like hunger, and describe the role learning plays in sexual attitudes and behavior.

2. Discuss the influence of culture on perceptions of "normal" and "abnormal" sexual orientations and practices.

3. Describe recent research findings on sexual attitudes, motives, and signals.

4. Explain how gender roles influence men's and women's sexual attitudes and behavior.

5. Describe various approaches to identifying and explaining different types/styles of love and discuss points upon which these theories agree.

Overview

This lesson deals with a wide range of intimate interactions between human beings, from attraction, affection, and love to sexual relations and lifelong attachment. It explains why psychologists debate over whether or not sex should be considered a primary drive like hunger or thirst. It shows why human sexuality is not as powerfully influenced by biological factors as are the procreative activities of most lower animals.

The lesson shows why learning plays such a critically important role in shaping human sexual attitudes and practices. It also examines the sociocultural factors that influence people's perceptions of what is "normal" and what is "abnormal" sexual behavior, including the perplexing problem of determining the origins of both **heterosexuality** and **homosexuality**. The lesson reports on research into **sexual attitudes**, **motives**, and **signals** and on why successful and satisfactory intimacy depends on each party understanding what the other means and intends.

Both the text and the video program show **gender roles** to be a significant force in determining how men and women think and feel about sex and love and how they behave toward one another. The lesson also examines the role played by **sexual scripts** in guiding the sexual behavior of young men and women and of adults.

The lesson describes several approaches to identifying and explaining different types or styles of **love** and loving. The theories of love examined include one that contrasts **passionate (romantic) love** with **companionate love**. Robert Sternberg's **triangle theory of love**, which considers love to consist of passion, intimacy, and commitment, is also described. The attachment theory of love and John Alan Lee's **theory of six styles of love**, an elegant and intricate categorization of what he calls the many "colors of love," are presented.

Viewing Notes

The video program "Gender and Relationships" helps explain why human emotional interactions and attachments are so complex.

Although we all have varying degrees of experience with affection, sexuality, love, and commitment, even the most respected authorities remain uncertain about what factors influence people's warmest feelings toward one another. The subjects covered in this lesson include some of the most beguiling mysteries of the ages: what is love; what makes sexual behavior "normal" or "abnormal"; and why and in what ways do men and women differ in their sexual attitudes, motives, and behavior? This video lesson provides some dramatic examples and illuminating explanations based on recent research.

As you watch the video program, consider the following questions:

1. Why and in what ways are close relationships changing in contemporary western society?

2. As explained by Carole Wade, how do men and boys differ from women and girls in their expectations about the nature of intimacy and closeness?

3. How does Jerald Jellison explain the exchange theory of interpersonal relations and especially what the theory considers "real" in a relationship?

4. What factors influence, and may even change, gender roles, gender identities, and gender stereotypes?

5. What does Anne Peplau say about the impact of norms, relative dependency, and resources in the "balance of power" in close relationships?

6. What do Alex and Grace Lopez say about how their marriage was affected by having children?

7. What does Warren Farrell, whose work is referred to by Martin Fiebert, mean when he says that men face far more risks when becoming involved in any relationship than women do?

8. In what ways do second marriages seem to differ from first marriages?

9. What are some of the factors that characterize successful, satisfying, and enduring relationships?

Review Exercises

Vocabulary Check

Match the following key terms and concepts with the appropriate definitions from the list below.

1. ___ attachment theory of love (pp. 427–428)

2. ___ companionate love (p. 426)

3. ___ exchange theory of interpersonal relations (video)

4. ___ gender identity (p. 513; video)

5. ___ gender role (p. 436; video)

6. ___ passionate (romantic) love (p. 426)

7. ___ sexual attitudes (pp. 436–438)

8. ___ sexual motives (pp. 434–436)

9. ___ sexual orientation (pp. 438–440)

10. ___ sexual scripts (pp. 436–437)

11. ___ sexual signals (p. 437)

12. ___ testosterone (p. 432)

13. ___ theory of six styles of love (p. 426; video)

14. ___ triangle theory of love (pp. 426–427)

a. how men and women feel about sexual behavior, whether they are conservative and idealistic or permissive and liberal about it

b. a set of norms that defines socially approved attitudes and behavior for men and women

c. what men and women consider the purpose of sexual activity (for instance, a physical act for pleasure or an emotional act for closeness)

d. John Alan Lee's categories or styles of loving, which he labeled with Greek names

e. the theory that what counts most in interpersonal relationships is not feelings, intentions, or desires, but behavior—what people actually do

f. term used to describe heterosexuality, homosexuality, and bisexuality

g. a hormone that may promote sexual desire in males and females

h. a kind of love characterized by a turmoil of intense emotions; the stuff of crushes, infatuations, "love at first sight," and the early stages of love affairs

i. relates adult styles of love to types of infant attachment

j. according to John Gagnon and William Simon, the guidelines that specify appropriate sexual behavior for a person in a given situation, varying according to the person's age, culture, and gender

k. Sternberg's idea that the ingredients of love are passion (butterflies in the stomach, euphoria, sexual excitement), intimacy (feeling free to talk about anything, being understanding and patient with the loved one), and commitment (needing one another, being loyal); in his view, varieties of love occur because of the ways people combine the three elements

l. one's sense of oneself as male or female

m. a kind of love characterized by affection and trust

n. what men and women say or do to get sex or love or to keep a companion

Other Key Terms and Concepts

contact comfort (p. 423)

gender schema (p. 514)

gender stereotypes (video)

gender typing (p. 514)

heterosexuality (p. 438)

homosexuality (p. 438)

love (pp. 426–428; video)

sociobiology (pp. 77–78)

Completion

Fill each blank with the most appropriate term from the list of answers below.

15. Biological factors, such as a minimum level of the sex hormone _____, may influence sexual desire in both men and women, but the greater role of _____ and _____ makes it hard to treat human sexuality as a primary drive like hunger.

16. Unlike most lower animals, human beings must _____ what they are supposed to do with their sexual desires, even how to have sexual relations.

17. Most people assume that their own sexual practices and preferences are _____.

18. No single theory can account for all the _____ of homosexuality and heterosexuality.

19. Even when the sexual _____ of men and women is alike, their sexual _____ often differ.

20. One basic distinction in types/styles of love is between _____ love and _____ love.

21. Some authorities believe that by adulthood, male sexuality has become _____ and _____, and that female sexuality in our society is more closely connected to _____.

22. _____ is an interdisciplinary field of study that looks for evolutionary explanations for social behavior in animals, including human beings.

23. As children mature, they develop a _____; that is, they begin to divide people into categories of male or female.

behavior	learn	passionate
companionate	learning	sociobiology
emotionally detached	love and attachment	sociocultural factors
gender schema	motives	testosterone
genitally focused	normal	varieties

True-False

Read the following statements carefully and mark each true (T) or false (F).

24. ___ Experts agree that sex is a primary drive like hunger.

25. ___ Sex researcher Leonore Tiefer maintains that, for human beings, "sex is not a natural act." People must learn from experience and cultural standards what they are supposed to do with their sexual desires.

26. ___ Kissing is so simple and natural that it is practiced in virtually every human society.

27. ___ Psychologists are quite certain why people within a given culture acquire the sexual preferences and passions they do.

28. ___ The theories of sociobiologists about human sexual behavior are so convincing that they have been subjected to little criticism.

29. ___ Research shows that college students, particularly young white women, seem to be under particular pressure to have unwanted sex.

30. ___ There are pressures on both sexes to conform to social rules regarding sexual behavior and attitudes.

31. ___ There are no points of agreement among the various theories of types/styles of love discussed in the text.

32. ___ Ludus and mania are just two of the psychological problems that can afflict people who are passionately in love.

33. ___ One theory of love is based on the idea that human beings have a basic need to form attachments to others.

34. ___ Exclusively psychological theories of the causes of homosexuality are supported by extensive research and documentation.

Short-Answer Questions

As a final review exercise, write brief answers to demonstrate that you are achieving the learning objectives of this lesson.

1. Explain why psychologists disagree over whether sex should be considered a primary drive like hunger, and describe the role learning plays in sexual attitudes and behavior.

2. Discuss the influence of culture on perceptions of "normal" and "abnormal" sexual orientations and practices.

3. Describe recent research findings on sexual attitudes, motives, and signals.

4. Explain how gender roles influence men's and women's sexual attitudes and behavior.

5. Describe various approaches to identifying and explaining different types/styles of love and discuss points upon which these theories agree.

Self-Test

1. Psychologists cannot agree that sex should be considered a primary drive or biological need, because

   a. many people can go for so long without sex.

   b. sex seems to be an innate drive only in males.

   c. human sexual behavior seems to depend not so much on an instinctual drive as on learning.

   d. virtually all animals must learn how to channel their sexual needs into appropriate sexual behavior.

2. Many different kinds of studies have implicated _____ as a principal biological factor influencing sexual motivation in both men and women

   a. genetic programming

   b. uncontrollable instincts

   c. the hormone estrogen

   d. the hormone testosterone

3. Human beings must learn

   a. that they should not make sexual overtures to a female when she is not in heat.

   b. that they should not become sexually active until approached by an experienced female.

   c. what they are supposed to do with their sexual desires: what is sexually stimulating, what parts of the body are erotic, and even how to engage in sexual relations.

   d. to suppress their sexual drive in the presence of more dominant males.

4. Sexual behavior takes place in a larger network of

   a. cultural norms, peers, and parental lessons.

   b. needs, drives, and appetites.

   c. learning and experience.

   d. irresistible impulses.

5. What is normal and correct sexual behavior
   a. is pretty much the same in all societies.
   b. varies greatly from one society to another.
   c. depends on the proportion of men to women in the society.
   d. depends on the age at which young people start to learn about sex.

6. The cause of homosexuality
   a. has been identified as genetic.
   b. is usually considered to be the influence of the homosexual's mother.
   c. is failed heterosexuality.
   d. involves an interaction of biology, culture, experiences, and opportunities; and, most important, may be different for different individuals.

7. For most people in close relationships, the primary motive for sexual relations is to
   a. have children.
   b. express love and intimacy and to experience erotic pleasure.
   c. demonstrate dominance.
   d. bind the other person to them.

8. The stereotype of the sexually promiscuous male and the coy and choosy female
   a. is common sense and undeniably accurate.
   b. often blinds people to greater evidence of the similarities between men and women in their need for attachment and love.
   c. has been verified by many researchers.
   d. is an invention of Hollywood scriptwriters.

9. Men and women _____ one another's sexual signals (or apparent sexual signals).

   a. are genetically programmed to understand

   b. usually have no trouble interpreting

   c. often misread

   d. seldom even notice

10. There is evidence that rape is

    a. usually an accidental phenomenon resulting from mutual overstimulation of sexually inexperienced individuals.

    b. almost exclusively committed by psychologically disordered sex offenders.

    c. primarily an act of dominance and aggression.

    d. typically a false accusation by a female wishing to harm or manipulate a sexual partner.

11. According to John Gagnon and William Simon, _____ teach boys and girls what to consider erotic or sexy and how to behave during dating and sex.

    a. older siblings and playmates

    b. parents and teachers

    c. sex therapists

    d. sexual scripts

12. Understanding that sexual attitudes and behavior are part of a larger pattern of _____ helps explain why men and women often approach sex in different ways.

    a. sexual drives

    b. gender roles

    c. social motives

    d. abnormal practices

13. Women who are most concerned with finding and keeping a secure relationship are likely to regard sex, consciously or unconsciously, as

    a. something to be enjoyed for its own sake.

    b. acceptable only if birth control is used.

    c. a bargaining chip.

    d. an activity to engage in aggressively and assertively.

14. Sandra is four years old. She likes dolls, pretty clothes, and jewelry and is passive and obedient—"a good little girl." Psychologists would say she is this way because she has been

    a. genetically programmed.

    b. gender identified.

    c. stereotyped.

    d. gender typed.

15. Which of the following does NOT characterize companionate love?

    a. a focus of one's life

    b. intense emotion

    c. not necessarily sexualized

    d. affection and trust

16. According to John Alan Lee's theory of styles of loving, which of the following is NOT one of the six basic styles?

    a. libido (sexually driven love)

    b. ludus (game-playing love)

    c. eros (romantic, passionate love)

    d. storge (affectionate, friendly love)

17. The one feature of love that seems to play a role in all the theories discussed in this lesson is

    a. romance.

    b. logic.

    c. attachment.

    d. devotion.

18. Cindy Hazan and Phillip Shaver believe that adult styles of love
    a. originate in early styles of infant-parent attachment.
    b. depend on each individual's sexual experience since puberty.
    c. are attributable to varying levels of sex hormones.
    d. are shaped by gender roles and social norms.

19. According to Sternberg's triangle theory, love consists of all the
    following factors EXCEPT
    a. intimacy.
    b. romance.
    c. passion.
    d. commitment.

Study Activities

The following activity challenges you to use your critical thinking and demonstrate how what you are learning can be applied to you and your own life. Try this activity and/or those your instructor assigns.

What is your style of loving? Review the coverage of different types and styles of love on pages 426–428 of the Wade and Tavris textbook, with special attention to John Alan Lee's six styles of love. You may also want to read Lee's book, *The Colours of Love* (Ontario, Canada: New Press, 1973).

Based on your reading and by examining your own experience, determine which of the styles characterize the way you have been in love at various times in your life. You probably will not have manifested only one style. The way you felt and acted when you first fell in love is unlikely to be identical to the way you love a dear old friend. Your love for a close relative will not resemble the passionate kind of love Lee refers to as mania. If you find Lee's categories are too refined, be guided by the other theories of love and decide if your general style of loving is more passionate than companionate, or more typified by attachment.

As you build some confidence with these concepts, try to apply them to people you have known—and perhaps loved. This activity can be of particular value and interest if you discover that someone you loved in one fashion may have loved you in quite another. The classic case, of course, is a person who loves another passionately or manically but is loved in return only in a playful or friendly manner. You may learn from this exercise that a romance was doomed from the beginning because your style of love and that of your loved one were in irreconcilable conflict. Conversely, romantic relationships that you have found to be satisfying and/or long-lasting may prove to have been strengthened and sustained by the fact that both parties had the same style of loving.

This analysis can be applied to people other than yourself. With careful and honest examination, you should be able to gain some insights into why couples of your acquaintance have been successful or unsuccessful in their love relationships.

Lesson 14

Theories of the Person and Personality

Assignments

For the most systematic coverage of this lesson, we suggest that you complete the assignments in the sequence listed below.

Before viewing the video program:

- Read the "Learning Objectives" and "Overview" for this lesson. Use the Learning Objectives to guide your reading, viewing, and thinking.

- Read the "Viewing Notes" for this lesson.

- Read Chapter 13, "Theories of Personality," pages 457–467, 475–482, and 485–492, in the Wade and Tavris text. First, familiarize yourself with its contents by reading the Chapter Outline. As you read, note terms and concepts set in bold or italic type, especially those defined in the margins. Take the Quick Quizzes to check your understanding of material being described and explained.

View the video program, "Personality"

After viewing the video program:

- Briefly note your answers to the questions at the end of the "Viewing Notes."

- Review all reading assignments for this lesson, including the Summary at the end of Chapter 13 in the textbook.

- Complete the "Review Exercises" to strengthen your understanding of this lesson's central concepts and terminology. Pay special attention to the "Vocabulary Check" exercise and the additional terms and concepts that follow—page references indicate where in the text assignment each term is defined. [Remember: there is a complete Glossary at the end of the text.]

- Take the "Self-Test" to measure the degree to which you are achieving this lesson's learning objectives. Check your answers against the "Answer Key" and review when necessary.

- Follow the suggestions in the "Study Activities" section at the end of this lesson and complete any other activities and projects assigned by your instructor.

Learning Objectives

When you have completed all assignments in this lesson, you should be able to:

1. Define personality and explain the importance of personality theories in the field of psychology.

2. Describe Freud's personality theory, including the concepts of the id, ego, and superego; explain the functions of defense mechanisms, giving several examples.

3. Describe Freud's psychosexual stages and his ideas about the role of the Oedipus complex and identification in personality development.

4. Explain ways in which the theories of Horney and Jung differ from traditional psychoanalytic theory.

5. Evaluate the influence and limitations of the psychoanalytic approach.

6. Describe and evaluate the key concepts of the behavioral and social-cognitive approaches to personality theory.

7. Describe and evaluate the key concepts of the humanist and existential approaches to personality theory.

8. Define "trait" and briefly summarize the contributions of "trait" theories to understanding personality development. In light of recent research, critique the trait approach to personality, especially in relation to the problems of consistency and predictability.

9. Describe the findings of recent research that suggests genes are involved in heritable aspects of personality such as temperaments.

10. Define and describe the characteristics of the private personality, the sense of self.

Overview

Most schools of psychology either have a theory of personality or have reasons for criticizing the theories of others. Personality is a popular subject with experts and laypersons alike. Because psychology concerns itself with how a person behaves, thinks, and feels, it seems obvious that psychologists should try to develop reliable descriptions of what a person really is, to discover the nature of personality.

The text and the video program define **personality** and explain its importance in psychology. They do so by introducing the major theories of personality developed by the various schools of psychology. The monumental, though highly controversial, formulations of Sigmund Freud are discussed in some detail. The **psychoanalytic theory of personality** is explained, including the concepts of the **id**, **ego**, and **superego**. The role of **defense mechanisms** is spelled out. Freud's **psychosexual stages of development** are outlined, including discussion of **identification** and the **Oedipus complex**.

This lesson discusses the ways in which some of Freud's followers—particularly Karen Horney and Carl Jung—departed from traditional psychoanalytic theory. The influence and limitations of Freud's theories are evaluated.

Behavioral psychologists' approach to personality and the personality theories of **social-cognitive theorists** and **humanist** and **existential psychologists** are examined and compared with one another and with the views of psychoanalytic theorists.

Many attempts have been made over the centuries to define universal personality qualities, traits, temperaments, or types. The lesson contrasts some of these with more scientific, modern **trait theory**, which may employ such methods as **factor analysis**. The textbook discusses recent research into the possible genetic basis of aspects of personality.

The concept of a **private personality**, a sense of self, is also considered. The lesson sheds some light on the controversial and still-unresolved problems of determining the degree to which personality is (or can be) stable, predictable, and consistent.

Viewing Notes

This video program examines various theories of personality and describes some of the current research that fuels these theories. Experts introduce major theories, such as the psychoanalytic, behavioral, social-learning, and humanist approaches. The program focuses on such "big questions" as "How do people get to be the way they are?" and "Does personality change, and if so, how?"

The role of trait theory is examined, and the importance of the interaction between the environment and personality characteristics is evaluated. Research into the biological foundations of personality is also introduced.

As you watch the video program, consider the following questions:

1. How is personality defined in the video program?

2. What does Richard Haier say are the principal objects and interests of people who study personality?

3. How do the various schools within the field of psychology approach the subject of human personality?

4. What are some of the attractive features of the psychoanalytic (or psychodynamic) theories of personality?

5. As explained by Lynn Carol Miller, what is the behavioral perspective on personality?

6. According to Salvatore Maddi, what do the humanists emphasize in their approach to personality?

7. What are some of the factors that Haier describes in explaining why modern trait theories of personality are more scientific than the many trait theories from earlier eras?

8. What does the video program show about the practical value of personality theories (such as the five-factor [Big Five] model of personality) based on factor analysis?

9. What does Haier say about the genetic components of personality traits and about his research into the biological mechanisms underlying personality?

10. What does Laura Baker say about the relative influences of shared and nonshared environments on personality development?

Review Exercises

Vocabulary Check

Match the following key terms and concepts with the appropriate definitions from the list below.

1. ___ collective unconscious (p. 481; video)

2. ___ defense mechanisms (p. 477; video)

3. ___ ego (p. 477; video)

4. ___ id (p. 476; video)

5. ___ personality (p. 458; video)

6. ___ private personality (p. 489)

7. ___ social-cognitive theories (pp. 466–467; video)

8. ___ temperaments (p. 463)

9. ___ trait (p. 458; video)

10. ___ unconditional positive regard (p. 488)

a.   a sense of self, an identity, through which we process and absorb experiences, thoughts, and emotions; an inner sense of continuity and perception

b.   characteristic styles of responding to the environment that appear in infancy or early childhood and are assumed to be innate

c.   to Carl Jung, the universal memories and experiences of humankind, represented in the unconscious of all people

d.   a descriptive characteristic of an individual, assumed to be stable across situations

e.   a distinctive and relatively stable pattern of behavior, thoughts, motives, and emotions that characterizes an individual

f.   in psychoanalysis, the part of the personality that represents reason, good sense, and rational self-control; operates according to the reality principle

g.   to Carl Rogers, love or support given to another person with no conditions attached

h.   in psychoanalysis, the part of the personality containing inherited psychological energy, particularly sexual and aggressive instincts; operates according to the pleasure principle

i.   theories that emphasize how personality traits are learned and maintained depending on the specific situation and the individual's cognitive processes

j. methods used by the ego to prevent unconscious anxiety from reaching consciousness

Other Key Terms and Concepts

archetypes (p. 481; video)

congruence (p. 487)

displacement (p. 478)

factor analysis (p. 459; video)

five-factor (Big Five) model of personality (pp. 459–460; video)

intrapsychic (p. 476)

inventories (p. 458)

libido (p. 476)

object-relations school (p. 482)

Oedipus complex (p. 479)

pleasure principle (p. 477)

psychoanalysis (p. 476; video)

psychodynamic theories (p. 476)

psychosexual stages (pp. 479–480; video)

reality principle (p. 477)

sublimation (p. 478)

superego (p. 477; video)

unconscious processes (pp. 476–477)

Completion

Fill each blank with the most appropriate term from the list of answers below.

11. Because psychology deals with the nature and meaning of a person's behavior, thoughts, motives, and emotions, many different _____ have been formulated to explain what a person is.

12. Sigmund Freud developed _____, which encompasses both a theory of personality and a method of psychotherapy.

13. Freud's theory and the approach of many of his followers is called _____, a word that refers to psychological theories that explain behavior in terms of forces located in the individual, such as inner drives, impulses, and motives, or, in psychoanalysis, instinctual energy.

14. The principal parts of the personality, according to Freud, are the _____, the _____, and the _____.

15. Repression, projection, and reaction formation are examples of _____.

16. Freud's psychosexual stages of personality development are, in order, the _____ stage, the _____ stage, the _____ stage, the _____ stage, and the _____ stage.

17. Carl Jung's greatest difference with Freud concerned the nature of the _____.

18. Among the many criticisms of psychoanalytic theory, one of the most damaging scientifically is that many of the ideas of Freud and his followers are little more than descriptive observations and poetic images that can't be _____ to confirm their validity.

19. Behaviorists, such as B. F. Skinner, have little interest in formulating theories of personality, because they see personality as a collection of _____ involving responses in certain situations.

20. According to _____, we acquire personality patterns as we learn to deal with the environment, and personality and situation are constantly influencing each other in an unending chain of interaction.

21. Abraham Maslow, Rollo May, and Carl Rogers have been the chief leaders among _____.

22. Gordon Allport is one of the most influential _____ of this century.

23. Researchers are finding that the private personality is made up of many _____, which might include the _____ self and the _____ self.

anal	ideal	real
behavioral patterns	latency	social-cognitive theories
defense mechanisms	oral	superego
ego	phallic (or Oedipal)	tested
genital	possible selves	theories of personality
humanist psychologists	psychoanalysis	trait theorists
id	psychodynamic	unconscious

True-False

Read the following statements carefully and mark each true (T) or false (F).

24. ___ Psychologists basically agree on which traits they consider the most important and in their views of the origins and stability of personality.

25. ___ Sigmund Freud considered conscious awareness only the tip of a mental iceberg, most of which was the vast, unrevealed unconscious part of the mind.

26. ___ According to Freud, the ego operates according to the pleasure principle.

27. ___ Those who employ projection as a defense mechanism attribute unacceptable feelings to someone else.

28. ___ Freud conceived the Oedipus complex (also termed the Electra complex when applied to female children) as a conflict in which a child desires the parent of the opposite sex and views the same-sex parent as a rival; Freud considered this the key issue in the phallic stage of development.

29. ___ Karen Horney and Carl Jung were among the few followers of Freud who loyally supported, defended, and tried to spread his ideas throughout their lives.

30. ___ Some critics of psychoanalysis felt Freud did not emphasize the unconscious enough, letting it be overshadowed by the importance of real events and conscious thoughts.

31. ___ Where behaviorists see personality as a set of habits and beliefs that have been rewarded over a person's lifetime, social-cognitive theorists maintain that these habits and beliefs eventually acquire a life of their own, coming to exert their own effects on behavior.

32. ___ According to humanist psychologist Carl Rogers, a fully functioning person shows congruence: harmony between the conscious self and the totality of the person's unconscious feelings and life experiences.

33. ___ The search for genes involved in heritable aspects of personality is preliminary, the findings are tentative, and there is little likelihood of it having much impact on future psychological study and theories.

34. ___ There is little debate over the idea that a person's personality is stable and unchanging throughout life.

Short-Answer Questions

As a final review exercise, write brief answers to demonstrate that you are achieving the learning objectives of this lesson.

1. Define personality and explain the importance of personality theories in the field of psychology.

2. Describe Freud's personality theory, including the concepts of the id, ego, and superego; explain the functions of defense mechanisms, giving several examples.

3. Describe Freud's psychosexual stages and his ideas about the role of the Oedipus complex and identification in personality development.

4. Explain ways in which the theories of Horney and Jung differ from traditional psychoanalytic theory.

5. Evaluate the influence and limitations of the psychoanalytic approach.

6. Describe and evaluate the key concepts of the behavioral and social-cognitive approaches to personality theory.

7. Describe and evaluate the key concepts of the humanist and existential approaches to personality theory.

8. Define "trait" and briefly summarize the contributions of trait theories to understanding personality development. In light of recent research, critique the trait approach to personality, especially in relation to the problems of consistency and predictability.

9. Describe the findings of recent research that suggests genes are involved in heritable aspects of personality such as temperaments.

10. Define and describe the characteristics of the private personality, the sense of self.

Self-Test

1. Personality is usually defined as a distinctive, relatively stable pattern of

    a. needs and drives.

    b. stimuli and responses.

    c. behavior, thoughts, motives, and emotions.

    d. physical characteristics, mannerisms, and attitudes.

2. Different schools of psychology analyze and define personality

    a. in much the same way.

    b. in several different ways.

    c. in ways based on Freud's classic formulation.

    d. only as a theoretical exercise.

3. Which of the following is **NOT** one of the three major systems in Freud's conception of the structure of personality?

    a. id

    b. ego

    c. libido

    d. superego

4. Which of the following defense mechanisms involves putting unacceptable feelings and thoughts into the unconscious?

    a. displacement

    b. denial

    c. repression

    d. projection

5. The _____ is the last element of Freud's system of personality to develop; it represents the voice of morality, the rules of parents and society, and the power of authority.

    a. ego

    b. superego

    c. ego ideal

    d. conscience

6. Which of Freud's psychosexual stages begins at puberty and marks the beginning of mature adult sexuality?

    a. anal stage

    b. genital stage

    c. oral stage

    d. latency stage

7. Which of the following identified universal, symbolic images that appear in myths, art, dreams, and other expressions of the collective unconscious?

    a. Freud

    b. Adler

    c. Jung

    d. Horney

8. Which of the following is **NOT** one of the problems critics have found with psychoanalysis?

    a. insufficiently imaginative

    b. untestable hypotheses

    c. overemphasis on unconscious processes rather than real experiences

    d. fallacy of generalizing to all human beings the insights gained from working with therapy patients

9. Contemporary researchers and clinical psychologists
   a. find little justification for drawing upon Freud's theories.

   b. are finding support for a few of Freud's assumptions.

   c. devote a great deal of time and effort to disproving psychoanalytic hypotheses.

   d. are mostly Freudians or neo-Freudians.

10. To behaviorists, _____ more important than personality in determining the causes of behavior.
    a. biological factors are

    b. the unconscious is

    c. the environment is

    d. the reality principle is

11. Which of the following is **NOT** one of the phenomena that social-cognitive theorists emphasize in their theories of personality?
    a. observational learning and the role of models

    b. cognitive processes such as perceptions and interpretations of events

    c. motivating beliefs

    d. unalterable genetic predispositions

12. Which of the following would humanist psychologists be **LEAST** likely to cite as one of the abilities that define human personality and separate us from other animals?
    a. free will

    b. inherited temperaments

    c. self-direction

    d. freedom of choice

13. The major criticism of humanist psychology is that
    a. it relies too much on biological factors.

    b. none of its leaders have clinical experience helping ordinary people.

    c. many of its assumptions cannot be tested because the terms humanists use are too vague.

    d. it is too objective and scientific, lacking a strong philosophical outlook.

14. Raymond B. Cattell advanced the study of personality traits by using a statistical method called
    a. locus of control.

    b. identification.

    c. factor analysis.

    d. phrenology.

15. The trait approach to personality
    a. demonstrates unusual consistency and predictability.

    b. removes the possibility of self-bias.

    c. is little more than a curiosity whose most important example is the ancient concept of typing people by which of their body fluids (humors) predominate.

    d. has been highly successful in identifying what seem to be the core dimensions or features that make one person different from another.

16. An important way to study the genetics of personality is to estimate the heritability of personality traits by
    a. testing the genetic material of all the children in families being studied.

    b. comparing a child's traits and temperament to those of his or her parents and grandparents.

    c. comparing a child's traits and temperament to those of an adopted sibling.

    d. comparing identical and fraternal twins reared apart with twins reared together.

17. Researchers believe they have found one of several genes involved in each of the following aspects of personality **EXCEPT**

    a.   neuroticism.

    b.   compassion.

    c.   pessimism.

    d.   anxiety.

18. The private personality reflects your interior sense of self, including the subjective experience of each of the following **EXCEPT**

    a.   emotions.

    b.   motivations.

    c.   memories.

    d.   wishes.

19. In addition to the private personality, each of us has _____

    a.   a biological personality.

    b.   an existential personality.

    c.   a public personality.

    d.   a social personality.

Study Activities

The following activity challenges you to use your critical thinking and demonstrate how what you are learning can be applied to you and your own life. Try this activity and/or those your instructor assigns.

What roles do personality and personality theory play in your life? Even if, until now, you have had little or no exposure to formal psychological theories of personality, you no doubt have been aware of the concept. You may have been told that you have a great personality, or a pleasant personality, or an abrasive personality—or no personality. You may have analyzed your feelings about other people in terms of their personalities, thinking that you like someone's personality or that he or she would be easier to get along with after a personality transplant.

Based on your study of this lesson, try to analyze your own personality and the personalities of people who are important in your life. Keeping in mind that efforts to characterize your own personality are almost always biased, submit your conclusions to as objective an evaluation as you can—and then reevaluate them. The purpose of this exercise is not to have you produce a definitive personality profile of yourself or anyone else. Experts, not to mention untrained phonies (see pages 491–492 in the Wade and Tavris textbook), have trouble doing that. What you should be doing is testing your growing knowledge of various personality theories by trying to apply some of the different concepts and categories to yourself and to people you know. It is more important, in this exercise, to see if you understand what the personality theorists are talking about than to worry about whether or not you are painting accurate personality portraits. Your existing knowledge of yourself and others, combined with your common sense, should keep you from going too far wrong. Your study of this lesson should prevent you from indulging in overgeneralization, oversimplification, and self-delusion.

Feel free to employ a personality theory that particularly appeals to you or to draw upon several theories. Use the exercise in any way that works for you, just as long as it gives you a chance to become familiar with the ideas and terminology of psychological approaches to personality.

Lesson 15

Measuring and Explaining
Human Diversity

Assignments

For the most systematic coverage of this lesson, we suggest that you complete the assignments in the sequence listed below.

Before viewing the video program:

- Read the "Learning Objectives" and "Overview" for this lesson. Use the Learning Objectives to guide your reading, viewing, and thinking.

- Read the "Viewing Notes" for this lesson.

- Read Chapter 2, "How Psychologists Do Research," pages 41–42; Chapter 3, "Evolution, Genes, and Behavior," pages 65–68, 80–83, and 89–94; and Chapter 9, "Thinking and Intelligence," pages 324–335. Also review Chapter 13, "Theories of Personality," pages 483–486, and Appendix, "Statistical Methods," pages A-4 to A-6, in the Wade and Tavris text. First, familiarize yourself with their contents by reading the Chapter Outlines. As you read, note terms and concepts set in bold or italic type, especially those defined in the margins. Take the Quick Quizzes to check your understanding of material being described and explained.

View the video program, "Intelligence"

After viewing the video program:

- Briefly note your answers to the questions at the end of the "Viewing Notes."

- Review all reading assignments for this lesson, including the Summaries at the end of Chapters 2, 3, 9, and 13 in the textbook.

- Complete the "Review Exercises" to strengthen your understanding of this lesson's central concepts and terminology. Pay special attention to the "Vocabulary Check" exercise and the additional terms and concepts that follow—page references indicate where in the text assignment each term is defined. [Remember: there is a complete Glossary at the end of the text.]

- Take the "Self-Test" to measure the degree to which you are achieving this lesson's learning objectives. Check your answers against the "Answer Key" and review when necessary.

- Follow the suggestions in the "Study Activities" section at the end of this lesson and complete any other activities and projects assigned by your instructor.

Learning Objectives

When you have completed all assignments in this lesson, you should be able to:

1. Define and explain the importance of reliability, validity, and standardization in test construction.

2. Discuss several different approaches to defining intelligence and explain why there is disagreement among psychologists on a single definition of intelligence.

3. Discuss in general terms what a typical intelligence test (IQ test) measures and provide examples of several mental skills and attributes it does not measure.

4. Explain how the normal (bell-shaped) curve and standard deviations are used to score intelligence tests.

5. Explain how an individual's cultural background may influence his or her performance on a psychological test.

6. Define and distinguish between various psychological assessment methods and discuss the usefulness and limitations of each approach.

7. Describe the controversy over the relative influence of genetic and environmental factors on mental ability.

8. Cite examples of the following eight environmental factors and explain how they may affect a child's mental ability: prenatal care, nutrition, exposure to toxins, mental stimulation, family size, individual experiences, stressful family circumstances, and parent-child interactions.

9. Discuss the predictive value and limitations of intelligence test scores.

Overview

This lesson, "Measuring and Explaining Human Diversity," deals largely with the ways psychologists define and measure human intelligence. The text and the video program make it clear that there is no one, agreed-upon definition of **intelligence**. They also show that what **intelligence (IQ) tests** can and cannot measure is the subject of considerable controversy and that psychologists have a wide variety of opinions on the utility of such tests.

Typical intelligence tests are described, and there is discussion of the need for **reliability**, **validity**, and **standardization** in test construction. The scoring of IQ tests, including the normal distribution (bell-shaped curve) and standard deviations, is explained.

The lesson gives considerable attention to the effect of an individual's cultural background on his or her performance on a psychological test. The video lesson covers the topic in terms of schoolchildren stigmatized as developmentally disabled and placed in special classes merely because English was not their native language and the IQ tests they took were really designed for those who speak English. The value of **culture-free** and **culture-fair tests** is discussed.

Various kinds of psychological assessment methods are described and evaluated, including **objective tests** and **projective tests**.

The nature-nurture issue, the controversy over the relative influence of genetic and environmental factors on mental ability, is carefully examined. No definitive answer is offered, but descriptions of recent research on the biological foundations of intelligence and on group differences in intelligence show the new questions and new possibilities raiseed by that research.

The lesson identifies environmental factors that may affect a child's mental development—both positively and negatively.

Finally, the predictive value and limitations of IQ test scores are discussed, explaining what current data now indicate about the correlation, if any, between IQ and success in school, occupation, creative endeavors, or just day-to-day living.

Viewing Notes

The video program for this lesson graphically demonstrates that there are significant differences between intellectually gifted individuals and those who are retarded or developmentally disabled. It also shows how hard it can be to define intelligence itself and to get experts to agree on what intelligence tests measure.

The program explains what intelligence tests are supposed to measure and what they probably can't measure. Historical film footage describes the origins of IQ tests, including some of the embarrassing failures of intelligence testing. Of particular interest is the debate over whether IQ tests measure aptitude (as they are supposed to do) or achievement (as their critics say they do). The issue is not settled, but strong arguments are presented for the idea that IQ tests primarily measure levels of learning, what knowledge individuals already possess, rather than their potential to learn.

As you watch the video program, consider the following questions:

1. What are some of the abilities that distinguish Justin, the gifted youngster, from Darryl, the little boy with Down's syndrome?

2. How do the different experts define intelligence?

3. Why does Jane Mercer say "intelligence" should be abolished from our vocabulary?

4. Can motivation, encouragement, and training increase a person's intellectual standing relative to other members of his or her peer group?

5. Does heredity play a significant role in intelligence?

6. What happens when children for whom English is not their native language are given IQ tests in English?

7. Under what circumstances can IQ tests provide useful information, and what are those sorts of information?

8. What does it mean to say IQs have a normal distribution, that they follow a bell-shaped curve?

9. What types of intellectual and cognitive abilities do IQ tests fail to measure?

10. What is the difference between an achievement test and an aptitude test?

11. Why does biological research using PET scanning of the brain suggest an efficiency model of intelligence?

12. Why is it that intelligence doesn't necessarily relate to achievement in life and that it is more important to make the most of what you are and what you have?

Review Exercises

Vocabulary Check

Match the following key terms and concepts with the appropriate definitions from the list below.

1. ___ achievement tests (p. 325; video)

2. ___ aptitude tests (p. 325; video)

3. ___ behavioral genetics (p. 81)

4. ___ culture-fair tests (pp. 329–330)

5. ___ culture-free tests (pp. 329–330)

6. ___ heritability (p. 81)

7. ___ intelligence (p. 324; video)

8. ___ intelligence quotient (IQ) (pp. 89, 325; video)

9. ___ monozygotic twins (identical twins) (p. 82)

10. ___ natural selection (p. 68)

11. ___ objective tests (inventories) (p. 41)

12. ___ projective tests (pp. 41, 483)

13. ___ psychometrics (p. 325)

14. ___ triarchic theory of intelligence (p. 330)

15. ___ validity (p. 42)

a. measurement of mental abilities, traits, and processes

b. twins born when a fertilized egg divides into two parts that develop into separate embryos

c. tests in which cultural experience does not influence performance

d. the evolutionary process in which individuals with genetically influenced traits that are adaptive in a particular environment tend to survive and to reproduce in greater numbers than do other individuals; as a result, their traits become more common in the population over time

e. Robert Sternberg's theory distinguishing three aspects of intelligence: componential, experiential, and contextual

f. tests designed to measure a person's potential for acquiring various types of skills and knowledge in the future

g. standardized objective questionnaires requiring answers or forcing choices

h. an inferred characteristic of an individual, usually defined as the ability to profit from experience, acquire knowledge, think abstractly, and adapt to changes in the environment

i. tests that reduce cultural bias by incorporating knowledge and skills common to many different cultures and socioeconomic groups

j. psychological tests used to infer a person's unconscious feelings or motives, thoughts, perceptions, and conflicts on the basis of the person's interpretations of ambiguous or unstructured stimuli

k. a test's ability to measure what it was designed to measure

l. tests designed to measure acquired skills and knowledge

m. a statistical estimate of the proportion of the total variance in a group of a trait that is attributable to genetic differences among individuals in the group

n. study of the genetic bases of individual differences in behavior and personality

o. a measure of intelligence originally computed by dividing a person's mental age by his or her chronological age and multiplying by 100

Other Key Terms and Concepts

chromosomes (p. 66)

Down's syndrome (video)

dizygotic twins (fraternal twins) (p. 82)

factor analysis (p. 324)

g factor (p. 324)

mental age (MA) (p. 325)

metacognition (p. 330)

normal distribution (bell-shaped or normal curve) (pp. 89, A-6)

norms (p. 41)

psychological tests (p. 41)

reliability (p. 41)

Rorschach Inkblot Test (p. 484)

standard deviation (p. A-4)

standardize (p. 41)

Completion

Fill each blank with the most appropriate term from the list of answers below.

16. The construction of good tests is reflected in _____, the consistency of scores derived from the test, _____, the ability of the test to measure what it was intended to measure, and _____, uniform procedures for giving the test and scoring it by referring to norms, or established standards of performance.

17. Among the many approaches to defining intelligence are those that distinguish between the ability to reason _____ and the ability to _____ from experience in daily life.

18. Mental tests may either be _____ tests, which are designed to measure acquired skills and knowledge, or _____ tests, which are supposed to measure a person's ability to acquire skills and knowledge in the future.

19. When large numbers of people take an IQ test, their scores tend to be distributed in a normal _____ curve, with scores near the average (mean) most common and very high or low scores rare.

20. Objective tests or _____ measure beliefs, feelings, or behaviors of which the individual is aware; _____ tests, such as the popular _____, are used to measure conscious and unconscious motives, thoughts, perceptions, and conflicts.

21. In the _____ debate over the relative influence of genetic and environmental factors on mental ability, studies of monozygotic, or _____, twins reared apart have provided some of the best clues to heritability, although critics have found _____ flaws in some of this research.

22. Whether or not you will enjoy occupational success can be predicted more accurately by considering your _____ and _____ rather than your IQ alone.

abstractly

achievement

aptitude

bell-shaped

education

identical

inventories

learn and profit

methodological

nature-nurture

projective

reliability

Rorschach Inkblot Test

socioeconomic background

standardization

validity

True-False

Read the following statements carefully and mark each true (T) or false (F).

23. ___ The validity of an intelligence test isn't as important as its reliability.

24. ___ Psychologists now agree that intelligence may best be defined as "whatever IQ tests measure."

25. ___ All mental tests are in some sense achievement tests because they assume some sort of past learning or experience with certain objects, words, or situations.

26. ___ Most mental tests do not measure experiential and contextual intelligence, what is sometimes called common sense or street smarts.

27. ___ In scoring IQ tests, the average (or mean) is arbitrarily set at 100 and a standard deviation determines how other scores spread out around the mean; as a result, most IQs come out above 100.

28. ___ An IQ test with questions which assume that those taking the test regularly read books and magazines could produce results that favor affluent people over the poor.

29. ___ Interviews are probably the most objective and reliable way to test intelligence or personality.

30. ___ Scientists are now able to determine the impact of heredity on any particular individual's intellectual or emotional makeup.

31. ___ Because lead has been banned from house paint, children's exposure to such toxins is no longer a threat to their mental development.

32. ___ The average gap between severely malnourished and well-nourished children can be as much as 20 IQ points.

33. ___ The idea that the environment influences IQ is supported by the fact that IQ scores in developed countries have been climbing for at least three generations, at a rate much too steep to be accounted for by genetic changes.

Short-Answer Questions

As a final review exercise, write brief answers to demonstrate that you are achieving the learning objectives of this lesson.

1. Define and explain the importance of reliability, validity, and standardization in test construction.

2. Discuss several different approaches to defining intelligence and explain why there is disagreement among psychologists on a single definition of intelligence.

3. Discuss in general terms what a typical intelligence test (IQ test) measures and provide examples of several mental skills and attributes it does not measure.

4. Explain how the normal (bell-shaped) curve and standard deviations are used to score intelligence tests.

5. Explain how an individual's cultural background may influence his or her performance on a psychological test.

6. Define and distinguish between various psychological assessment methods and discuss the usefulness and limitations of each approach.

7. Describe the controversy over the relative influence of genetic and environmental factors on mental ability.

8. Cite examples of the following eight environmental factors and explain how they may affect a child's mental ability: prenatal care, nutrition, exposure to toxins, mental stimulation, family size, individual experiences, stressful family circumstances, and parent-child interactions.

9. Discuss the predictive value and limitations of intelligence test scores.

Self-Test

1. Any good test (including any good IQ test) must be both
   a. valid and reliable.

   b. objective and projective.

   c. a measure of aptitude and a measure of achievement.

   d. monozygotic and dizygotic.

2. The norms, or established standards of performance, in a standardized test are developed by
   a. panels of expert psychometricians who evaluate each question for validity and reliability.

   b. community groups who judge if the test is culture-fair and culture-free.

   c. giving the test to a large group of people with characteristics similar to those for whom the test is intended.

   d. following regulations provided by government departments of education.

3. Which of the following has **NOT** been among the factors that have been considered by the many theorists who have tried to define intelligence?
   a. the ability to think rationally and reason abstractly

   b. the ability to make the most of what capacities one has

   c. the ability to learn and profit from experience

   d. the ability to act purposefully

4. Which of the following is **NOT** one of the aspects of intelligence in Robert Sternberg's triarchic theory of intelligence?
   a. componential intelligence

   b. experiential intelligence

   c. contextual intelligence

   d. standardized intelligence

5. Which of the following is the MOST likely reason psychologists cannot agree on a single definition of intelligence?

    a. Intelligence will never be defined until the nature-nurture issue is settled.

    b. Intelligence is a highly complex, multifaceted concept that encourages experts to consider it from different and sometimes conflicting perspectives.

    c. No one since Alfred Binet has thoroughly understood how to make IQ tests reveal the true nature of intelligence.

    d. Most theorists seem to focus on the differences between their ideas and those of other experts, rather than acknowledging similarities that might lead to a single comprehensive definition.

6. Most experts agree that IQ tests should measure _____, but most actually measure _____.

    a. achievement; aptitude

    b. aptitude; achievement

    c. aptitude; personality

    d. experience; heredity

7. Traditional intelligence tests are WEAKEST in their ability to measure

    a. how well a person can remember.

    b. whether or not a person can reason analytically.

    c. if a person can modify his or her behavior to adapt to different environments.

    d. how much a person has learned in school and elsewhere.

8. If the scores in large populations of people taking an IQ test are charted, they are expected to be distributed in a normal (bell-shaped) curve, with

    a. most scores falling above 100.

    b. few scores falling below 100.

    c. about two-thirds of the scores falling at exactly 100.

    d. about two-thirds of the scores falling between 85 and 115.

9. In a normal distribution of IQ test scores, one should expect to find that there are

    a. more IQs below 85 than above 115.

    b. more IQs above 115 than below 85.

    c. more IQs below 85 and above 115 combined than between 85 and 115.

    d. about the same number of scores below 85 as there are above 115.

10. Why did many European immigrants to the United States who were given intelligence tests early in the twentieth century get low scores, although many of their descendants later tested very high in IQ?

    a. The immigrants were genetically low in intelligence.

    b. The tests included many questions only people with long exposure to American culture and language could have answered.

    c. The immigrants hadn't taken such tests before, and so lacked the experience necessary to get a good score.

    d. The descendants were the products of marriages between immigrants and Americans with higher IQs.

11. Tests in which cultural experience does not influence performance are known as _____ tests.

    a. objective

    b. culture-fair

    c. culture-free

    d. projective

12. _____ tests, also called "inventories," measure beliefs, feelings, or behaviors of which an individual is aware.

    a. Objective

    b. Projective

    c. Aptitude

    d. Achievement

13. Which of the following aspects in scoring the Rorschach Inkblot Test is interpreted subjectively by most clinicians?

    a.   artistic merit

    b.   meaning

    c.   originality

    d.   content

14. The projective test that consists of a series of symmetrical abstract patterns is called the

    a.   Stanford-Binet Intelligence Test.

    b.   Rorschach Inkblot Test.

    c.   Minnesota Multiphasic Personality Inventory (MMPI).

    d.   Wechsler Adult Intelligence Scale-Revised (WAIS-R).

15. Which of the following is **NOT** true of heritable traits?

    a.   Heritability estimates do not apply to individuals, only to groups.

    b.   Not all traits you are born with are inherited.

    c.   They can be modified by the environment.

    d.   Heritability doesn't change over time.

16. It is fair to say that the available data _____ racial differences in IQ.

    a.   support a genetic explanation of

    b.   fail to support a genetic explanation of

    c.   indicate that environmental factors alone explain

    d.   prove that inadequacies in intelligence testing cause

17. Research on the biological foundations of intelligence has
    a. failed to locate any area or structure in the brain that seems to be associated with intelligent behavior or abstract reasoning.
    b. located areas of the brain that seem to be associated with intelligent behavior or abstract reasoning.
    c. thus far only determined that the brain cannot distinguish aptitude from achievement.
    d. shown that the people who did best on tests used the least amount of glucose energy, indicating an efficiency model of the brain.

18. Research has shown that a healthy and stimulating childhood environment
    a. can increase an individual's IQ by 15 to 30 points.
    b. produces statistically insignificant changes in IQ.
    c. raises the IQ of only those individuals whose parents have high IQs.
    d. can increase IQ, but only by a trivial 2 to 5 points.

19. In general, children who score well on IQ tests have parents who
    a. pay for tutors and special schools.
    b. have very high IQs.
    c. punish them if they fail to do well.
    d. spend time with them and actively encourage their development.

20. IQ scores are best at predicting performance in
    a. school.
    b. creative and artistic activities.
    c. occupational endeavors.
    d. day-to-day life.

21. The success of even gifted people is probably as attributable to having
_____ as to having a high IQ.

    a.   things made easy for them

    b.   drive, determination, and dedication

    c.   little competition

    d.   a great deal of luck

Study Activities

The following activity challenges you to use your critical thinking and demonstrate how what you are learning can be applied to you and your own life. Try this activity and/or those your instructor assigns.

Think about all the ways your aptitudes and achievements have been measured throughout your life. Starting with your earliest recollections, make a list of all the occasions on which your characteristics, attributes, skills, abilities, and accomplishments have been tested, measured, or compared to those of others. In a sense, your participation in the measuring and explaining of human diversity began at your birth. Soon after you began to breathe, you were weighed and your length was measured. When your parents were questioned about their new offspring—you—their first comments almost certainly included a statement such as "The baby weighed 7 pounds, 10 ounces." For the rest of your life, you have been and will be measured and evaluated.

The purpose of this study activity is to make you aware of the scope of this evaluation process, which is so widespread and pervasive in modern society. So much testing and measuring goes on that most people don't even notice or think about it. In fact, this exercise may remind you of long-forgotten tests you've taken and call attention to times you've been evaluated that didn't seem like tests when you experienced them.

Everyone remembers taking tests in school. As you make your list of testing experiences, you don't have to include every spelling test, recitation of the multiplication tables, and the like. You may mention all the kinds of tests you took in various grades. You certainly should indicate any special forms of evaluation to which you were subjected. Did you, for example, undergo any admissions tests or interviews at any level of your education, including private or special school admissions and college admissions? Did you take any college entrance examinations? Do you remember taking IQ tests, personality tests, vocational interest inventories, or any standardized tests purporting to determine the kind of person you were and what form your aptitudes took? Outside of educational settings, did you have to take any tests to get a job or a promotion? Have you taken any psychological tests, such as the Rorschach Inkblot Test or the Thematic Apperception Test (TAT), designed to reveal your feelings or thoughts?

You undoubtedly get the idea of this exercise. Guided by these examples and the material in the lesson, examine your recollections and try to produce a comprehensive list of the kinds of tests you've taken. Make a special effort to identify experiences that may not have seemed like tests at the time, such as one-to-one interviews where the other party seemed to have all the questions memorized and may have been taking notes after each of your responses. If you wish, you may list physical tests as well, which could include everything from medical examinations to sports contests in which your performance was timed, measured, and compared to that of others. Make your record as complete as you need it to be to understand that testing goes on all the time and virtually no one goes untested.

Lesson 16

Child Development

Assignments

For the most systematic coverage of this lesson, we suggest that you complete the assignments in the sequence listed below.

Before viewing the video program:

- Read the "Learning Objectives" and "Overview" for this lesson. Use the Learning Objectives to guide your reading, viewing, and thinking.

- Read the "Viewing Notes" for this lesson.

- Read Chapter 14, "Development over the Life Span," pages 497–504, 505–510, and 513–517, and Chapter 12, "Motivation," pages 422–425, in the Wade and Tavris text. First, familiarize yourself with their contents by reading the Chapter Outlines. As you read, note terms and concepts set in bold or italic type, especially those defined in the margins. Take the Quick Quizzes to check your understanding of material being described and explained.

View the video program, "Cognitive Development"

After viewing the video program:

- Briefly note your answers to the questions at the end of the "Viewing Notes."

- Review all reading assignments for this lesson, including the Summaries at the end of Chapters 14 and 12 in the textbook.

- Complete the "Review Exercises" to strengthen your understanding of this lesson's central concepts and terminology. Pay special attention to the "Vocabulary Check" exercise and the additional terms and concepts that follow—page references indicate where in the text assignment each term is defined. [Remember: there is a complete Glossary at the end of the text.]

- Take the "Self-Test" to measure the degree to which you are achieving this lesson's learning objectives. Check your answers against the "Answer Key" and review when necessary.

- Follow the suggestions in the "Study Activities" section at the end of this lesson and complete any other activities and projects assigned by your instructor.

Learning Objectives

When you have completed all assignments in this lesson, you should be able to:

1. Cite several examples of key child-development processes studied by psychologists; explain the importance of studying universal aspects of development as well as cultural and individual differences; and be aware that some psychologists view development as a series of distinct stages and others think of development as a series of small, gradual, continuous steps that blend into each other.

2. Identify several factors that can be harmful to the developing fetus.

3. Describe the reflexes and perceptual skills of newborns, and identify some of the developmental milestones usually achieved in the first year.

4. Explain Jean Piaget's view of cognitive development in children and discuss the processes of organization, adaptation, assimilation, and accommodation.

5. Name and describe Piaget's four stages of cognitive development: sensorimotor stage (birth to age 2), preoperational stage (ages 2 to 7), concrete operations stage (ages 6 or 7 to 11), and formal operations stage (ages 12 to adulthood).

6. Identify several problems researchers have found with Piaget's theory and discuss pros and cons related to trying to speed up children's cognitive development—what Piaget called "the American question."

7. Define attachment and explain its importance to a child's social development.

8. Explain the roles that gender typing and gender identity play in the development of each child's sense of self.

Overview

This lesson describes some of the key child-development processes that psychologists study. It explains that there are universal, individual, and cultural differences in development and that there is an ongoing controversy over whether development proceeds through stages or as a series of discrete but continuous steps.

Prenatal development is described, with special attention to several factors that can be harmful to the developing fetus, including smoking, drinking, drugs, German measles (rubella), X rays or other radiation, toxic chemicals, and sexually transmitted diseases. The developmental milestones of the first year of life are charted.

A large part of the text assignment and most of the video program concern cognitive development and particularly the theories of Jean Piaget. His concepts of **organization**, **adaptation**, **assimilation**, and **accommodation** are discussed. Piaget's four stages of cognitive development—**sensorimotor**, **preoperational**, **concrete operations**, and **formal operations**—are delineated. Critical aspects of passage through these stages are illustrated in the text and video lesson, including the concepts of **object permanence** and of **conservation**. The lesson also addresses the issue of accelerating the "natural" pace of development.

Criticisms of Piaget's ideas are presented and evaluated. Experts appearing in the video program and commentary in the text provide students ample opportunity to decide whether Piaget's theories are largely valid or generally flawed.

The importance of **attachment** to a child's social development is demonstrated, including video coverage of the interaction of emotional and cognitive development.

The lesson also explains the roles of **gender typing** and **gender identity** in the process of developing a child's sense of self.

Viewing Notes

Cognitive development is perhaps the most significant aspect of child psychology. Consequently, for this lesson, the video program is devoted almost entirely to cognitive development. The program focuses on the extremely influential theories of Jean Piaget. His concept of stages of cognitive development is described and explained, with dramatic demonstrations of children's cognitive skills at different stages.

Several experts discuss how children's ability to think, reason, remember, and use language develop. They comment on the value of Piaget's theories, acknowledging his impact on the field of child psychology, recognizing his lasting contributions, and identifying aspects of his work that subsequent research has called into question.

The video lesson also demonstrates that cognitive development is influenced by cultural factors and that it depends on emotion and social interaction.

As you watch the video program, consider the following questions:

1. What does Harold Chipman mean when he says "children actually think rather differently than we do. They are not just simplified adults. They really have thought processes of their own"?

2. How does Patricia Greenfield describe Piaget's four stages of cognitive development?

3. How does the use of language and symbols figure in a child's movement to higher stages of cognitive development?

4. Are the experiments concerning object permanence and conservation convincing proofs of Piaget's theories?

5. What criticisms of Piaget's ideas seem to have the most validity?

6. What was Piaget's position on trying to accelerate the pace of cognitive development?

7. Do the cognitive skills of the New Guinea children seem fundamentally different from those of the Western children in the program?

8. What makes sensitive parenting different and valuable?

Review Exercises

Vocabulary Check

Match the following key terms and concepts with the appropriate definitions from the list below.

1. ___ accommodation (p. 505)
2. ___ assimilation (p. 505)
3. ___ attachment (p. 422; video)
4. ___ concrete operations stage (p. 507; video)
5. ___ conservation (p. 506; video)
6. ___ egocentric thinking (p. 506)
7. ___ fetal alcohol syndrome (FAS) (p. 499)
8. ___ gender identity (p. 513)
9. ___ gender typing (gender socialization) (p. 514)
10. ___ object permanence (p. 506; video)
11. ___ operations (p. 506; video)
12. ___ preoperational (prelogical) stage (p. 506; video)
13. ___ reflexes (p. 500)
14. ___ synchrony (p. 501)

a. the third of Piaget's stages of cognitive development, during which the child can perform mental operations, explain these mental transformations, and solve problems imaginatively, but not in systematic or entirely logical ways

b. the understanding that an object continues to exist even when you can't see or touch it

c. a strong emotional tie between babies and their primary caretakers

d. the process of absorbing new information into existing cognitive structures, modifying it to "fit," if necessary

e. perceiving the world only from one's own point of view; the inability to take another person's perspective

f. the adjustment of one person's nonverbal behavior to coordinate with another's

g. the sense of being male or female, whether or not one follows the rules of gender typing

h. in Piaget's theory, mental actions that are cognitively reversible

i.   a pattern of physical and intellectual abnormalities in infants whose mothers drank more than two alcoholic drinks per day during pregnancy

j.   automatic behaviors that are necessary for survival

k.   the process by which children learn the behaviors, attitudes, and expectations associated in their culture with being "masculine" or "feminine"

l.   the understanding that the physical properties of objects—such as number of items, amount of liquid, or length of an object—remain the same even when appearances change (as long as nothing is added or taken away)

m.   Piaget's second stage of cognitive development, when the child gains the capacity for representational thought, using symbols and language, but cannot understand abstract principles or cause and effect

n.   the process of modifying existing cognitive structures in response to experience and new information

Other Key Terms and Concepts

contact comfort (p. 423)

formal operations stage (p. 507; video)

maturation (p. 498)

sensitive parenting (video)

sensorimotor stage (p. 506; video)

separation anxiety (p. 423)

socialization (p. 498)

theory of mind (p. 509)

Completion

Fill each blank with the most appropriate term from the list of answers below.

15.   Child psychologists study many facets of a child's _____, _____, _____, and _____ development.

16.   Among the factors that can be harmful to the developing fetus are _____, _____, _____, and _____.

17.   The reflexes of newborn babies include _____ and _____.

18.   Jean Piaget proposed that mental functioning depends on two basic biological processes: _____ and _____.

19. The first of Piaget's stages of cognitive development is called the _____ stage, during which the baby's major accomplishment is _____, the understanding that something continues to exist even if you can no longer see or touch it.

20. Americans visiting Piaget so often asked him about _____ child development, he referred to that query as "the American question."

21. Although Piaget's theories have been generally respected and widely influential, critics have identified many problems with his stage theory in general and with several specific aspects of it; a particularly significant criticism has been that changes, such as from _____ thought to _____ thought, are neither as clear-cut nor as sweeping as Piaget implied.

22. _____ is the innate need, in primate infants, for close physical contact; it is the basis of an infant's first attachment.

23. Girls believing they are supposed to like cooking and playing house and boys feeling they should want to engage in competitive sports are probably the result of _____, whereas their sense of being female or male is attributable to _____.

adaptation	gender typing	preoperational
alcohol	German measles (rubella)	sensorimotor
cigarettes	grasping	sexually transmitted diseases
cognitive	moral	
concrete operational	object permanence	social
contact comfort	organization	speeding up
gender identity	physical	sucking

True-False

Read the following statements carefully and mark each true (T) or false (F).

24. ____ Most psychologists study universal aspects of child development and are interested in individual differences in development, but few take cultural differences into account.

25. ____ Sexually transmitted diseases, such as syphilis, can cause mental retardation, blindness, and other physical disorders in the newborn, and, in the case of AIDS, an early death.

26. ____ Visual ability develops very slowly in newborns.

27. ____ Accommodation is the process of modifying your existing understanding.

28. ____ Piaget's four stages of cognitive development are, in order, preoperational, formal operations, concrete operations, and sensorimotor.

29. ____ Piaget felt that children's cognitive development should be accelerated as much as each child's abilities permit.

30. ____ Research has shown that so-called preoperational children can understand more than Piaget gave them credit for.

31. ____ Unlike adults, children do not have a "theory of mind"; that is, they lack a theory about how their own minds or other people's minds work and how people are affected by their beliefs and feelings.

32. ____ Everyone agrees that attachment, the strong emotional tie between babies and their primary caretakers, is important and that if infants are deprived of social contact, affection, and cuddling, the negative effects can be long-lasting.

33. ____ In contemporary Western society, gender typing and gender identity now apply almost exclusively to female children.

Short-Answer Questions

As a final review exercise, write brief answers to demonstrate that you are achieving the learning objectives of this lesson.

1. Cite several examples of key child-development processes studied by psychologists; explain the importance of studying universal aspects of development as well as cultural and individual differences; and be aware that some psychologists view development as a series of distinct stages and others think of development as a series of small, gradual, continuous steps that blend into each other.

2. Identify several factors that can be harmful to the developing fetus.

3. Describe the reflexes and perceptual skills of newborns, and identify some of the developmental milestones usually achieved in the first year.

4. Explain Jean Piaget's view of cognitive development in children and discuss the processes of organization, adaptation, assimilation, and accommodation.

5. Describe Piaget's four stages of cognitive development: sensorimotor stage (birth to age 2), preoperational stage (ages 2 to 7), concrete operations stage (ages 6 or 7 to 11), and formal operations stage (ages 12 to adulthood).

6. Identify several problems researchers have found with Piaget's theory and discuss pros and cons related to trying to speed up children's cognitive development—what Piaget called "the American question."

7. Define attachment and explain its importance to a child's social development.

8. Explain the roles that gender typing and gender identity play in the development of each child's sense of self.

Self-Test

1. A process of interest to developmental psychologists is _____, the sequential unfolding of genetically governed behavior and physical characteristics.

   a. maturation

   b. accommodation

   c. assimilation

   d. adaptation

2. Which of the following is **NOT** one of the aspects of development studied by psychologists?

   a. universal aspects of development

   b. individual differences in development

   c. cultural differences in development

   d. immutable laws of development

3. Kimberly's mother regularly drank large quantities of alcoholic beverages during her pregnancy. As an infant, Kimberly had a small brain and was uncoordinated, and now she shows signs of mental retardation. It is most likely that Kimberly is suffering from

   a. rubella (German measles).

   b. fetal alcohol syndrome.

   c. sudden infant death syndrome.

   d. teratogen embryosis.

4. Which of the following would contribute **LEAST** to helping a pregnant woman protect her developing fetus?

   a. quitting smoking

   b. taking no drugs unless they are medically necessary and tested for safety

   c. drinking little or no alcohol

   d. maintaining a low-fat, high-fiber diet

5. Newborn babies do **NOT** have which of the following reflexes?
    a. sucking

    b. reaching

    c. grasping

    d. rooting

6. Newborns are _____ from the first; they have inborn abilities to _____.

    a. irritable; annoy all adults and older children who approach them

    b. introverted; remain quiet or asleep while growing and developing strength and confidence

    c. sociable; attract adults to care for them

    d. aware; recognize the people and events around them

7. Which of the following are **NOT** among the developmental milestones reached by most children before the end of their first year of life?

    a. crawling, or walking with support

    b. saying first meaningful words

    c. beginning to solve problems logically

    d. communicating emotions through facial expressions

8. Cognitive development, according to Piaget's theory,

    a. is a series of small, gradual, continuous steps that blend into one another.

    b. involves four stages, which may be achieved at different ages but follow a fixed order, with each building on the one before.

    c. involves four stages experienced in an order that depends on each child's natural ability and rate of learning.

    d. involves four stages, all of which only the brightest children attain.

9. A child who knows that the family's Great Dane is a dog, but who has never seen a horse, may call the horse "doggie." This is an instance of what Piaget called

    a. adaptation.

    b. organization.

    c. accommodation.

    d. assimilation.

10. Babies start to understand the concept of object permanence, that something that is out of sight still exists, during the stage of cognitive development Piaget called the _____ stage.

    a. sensorimotor

    b. preoperational

    c. concrete operations

    d. formal operations

11. The accelerated use of symbols and language is the essential aspect of the _____ stage.

    a. sensorimotor

    b. preoperational

    c. concrete operations

    d. formal operations

12. If Piaget's theory is correct, adults should have passed through the three preceding stages and their cognitive development should be at the _____ stage.

    a. sensorimotor

    b. preoperational

    c. concrete operations

    d. formal operations

13. Researchers testing Piaget's theory of object permanence have found evidence that children who do not understand this concept

    a. are probably being pushed too fast by their parents.

    b. may not have a problem with undeveloped cognitive abilities in general so much as some difficulty with memory or an inability to reach for the objects.

    c. were not making themselves clear enough when speaking to adults about the missing object.

    d. may not have had enough practice.

14. Piaget's theory of object permanence has been criticized because

    a. even some adults lack this concept.

    b. researchers have found that the concept is mastered at a later stage than Piaget indicated.

    c. babies in Piaget's test were caught up in the peek-a-boo games and tried to fool Piaget and his colleagues.

    d. his tests were conducted using inanimate objects, ignoring the fact that young children have a good sense of "person permanence."

15. Research has shown that children _____ Piaget gave them credit for.

    a. understand far less than

    b. understand more than

    c. are incapable of understanding as much as

    d. require early enrichment to understand as much as

16. Piaget's answer to the question: "How can you speed up development?" was to

    a. encourage any efforts that might make children improve their cognitive skills.

    b. point out that accelerating development was virtually impossible.

    c. indicate that it made little sense to go beyond what is natural to a child of any given age and that such efforts would probably be detrimental to the child.

    d. provide detailed instructional exercises to accelerate cognitive development.

17. A baby will **NOT** develop well in a caretaking arrangement in which _____ is(are) absent.

    a. attachment

    b. his or her natural mother

    c. other children

    d. early enrichment

18. Parents and teachers can help children perform at a higher level than they could alone by providing _____, which helps a child carry out successively more complex acts and sustain the ones he or she is already able to perform.

    a. enrichment

    b. bonding

    c. scaffolding

    d. attachment

19. Only little girls lacking gender identity would

    a. play with toy soldiers.

    b. not think of themselves as being biologically female.

    c. be aggressive and competitive.

    d. prefer to wear pants and shirts instead of dresses.

20. Gender typing usually begins

    a. early in a child's life.

    b. when a child is in school with children of both sexes.

    c. with puberty.

    d. with dating and courtship.

Study Activities

The following activity challenges you to use your critical thinking and demonstrate how what you are learning can be applied to you and your own life. Try this activity and/or those your instructor assigns.

You must have noticed that much of both the text assignment and the video program deal with Jean Piaget's theories of cognitive development and with criticisms of his ideas. Clearly, his concepts are of critical importance in the subject of child development. Based on what you have already learned and on additional reading you may want to do of Piaget's works and those of his critics, you should be able to perform the following informal study.

See for yourself if Piaget's theories of object permanence and conservation actually work. If you have young children of your own, you can test the concepts on them. To test the concepts fully and fairly, however, you'll need children of different ages, so unless you have a very large family, you may have to get assistance from other parents. You might ask relatives or friends to let you test their children. If that approach is unrealistic, you can contact local nurseries, day-care centers, and elementary schools. Explain that you are a student of psychology and would appreciate their cooperation in your efforts to learn more about child development. They may well be eager to accommodate your request and may even volunteer to assist you, being interested themselves in the outcome of such tests.

Before you arrange for a time and place to test the children, be sure you have outlined exactly how you will perform the tests. Several of Piaget's works and books on Piaget, as well as texts on cognitive development or child development (see the bibliography in the Wade and Tavris textbook), have fairly detailed descriptions of how the studies of object permanence and conservation are performed. Follow those guidelines, providing yourself with a written plan you have rehearsed several times before doing your actual performance with children.

While doing the tests, go slowly and patiently, observing carefully and recording your observations as soon as possible after completing each test. When you have tested several children of appropriate ages for each concept, analyze your data to see if Piaget's ideas are, for the most part, generally correct or if his critics have a point.

Finally, as a personal check on Piaget, ask yourself if, while selecting a glass for some beverage, you ever choose a taller one when you're particularly thirsty, even though a shorter, wider one might, if you checked it as in the conservation experiment, actually hold more liquid.

Lesson 17

Later Childhood and Adolescence

Assignments

For the most systematic coverage of this lesson, we suggest that you complete the assignments in the sequence listed below.

Before viewing the video program:

- Read the "Learning Objectives" and "Overview" for this lesson. Use the Learning Objectives to guide your reading, viewing, and thinking.

- Read the "Viewing Notes" for this lesson.

- Read Chapter 14, "Development over the Life Span," pages 510–512, 518–527, and 537–538, and review pages 505–509 in the Wade and Tavris text. First, familiarize yourself with its contents by reading the Chapter Outline. As you read, note terms and concepts set in bold or italic type, especially those defined in the margins. Take the Quick Quizzes to check your understanding of material being described and explained.

View the video program, "Adolescent Development"

After viewing the video program:

- Briefly note your answers to the questions at the end of the "Viewing Notes."

- Review all reading assignments for this lesson, including the Summary at the end of Chapter 14 in the textbook.

- Complete the "Review Exercises" to strengthen your understanding of this lesson's central concepts and terminology. Pay special attention to the "Vocabulary Check" exercise and the additional terms and concepts that follow—page references indicate where in the text assignment each term is defined. [Remember: there is a complete Glossary at the end of the text.]

- Take the "Self-Test" to measure the degree to which you are achieving this lesson's learning objectives. Check your answers against the "Answer Key" and review when necessary.

- Follow the suggestions in the "Study Activities" section at the end of this lesson and complete any other activities and projects assigned by your instructor.

Learning Objectives

When you have completed all assignments in this lesson, you should be able to:

1. Describe and distinguish between the induction method of child rearing and power-assertion methods, and discuss the possible effects of each on the child.

2. Briefly describe Kohlberg's theory of moral development and discuss several criticisms of his theory.

3. Discuss the effect of childhood experience on the adult and discuss the implications of cases in which adults have overcome difficult childhoods.

4. Describe changes produced by hormones during puberty.

5. Describe intellectual development during adolescence.

6. Identify several factors that may help or hinder adolescents' ability to deal with the transition to adulthood.

Overview

This lesson begins with an examination of the two basic approaches to child rearing—the **induction method** and **power-assertions methods**—and of the different ways they affect the developing child. The importance to the child of interaction with peers and siblings is considered.

Children's moral development is explained, concentrating on the highly influential theories of Lawrence Kohlberg. The **stages of moral reasoning** that are the basis of his concept are described, and criticisms of his ideas are presented. There is also discussion of the development of conscience, which depends on **empathy**.

The effect of childhood experience on the adult is explored, with special attention to children's capacity to cope with and overcome traumatic childhoods marked by such problems as parental alcoholism and abuse.

The preponderance of the video lesson and a large part of the text assignment are devoted to the all-important transition from **adolescence** to adulthood. They clearly explain the physical changes, caused by hormones, that characterize biological **puberty**. They discuss the psychological upheavals accompanying adolescence and describe aspects of intellectual development in the teen years.

Because adolescence can be such a difficult time for many young people, the lesson carefully considers the factors that may help or hinder teenagers in their efforts to deal with the transition to adulthood.

Viewing Notes

The video program for this lesson, "Adolescent Development," captures some of the special flavor of that time during which exciting physical, social, and psychological changes force individuals to make the transition from childhood to adulthood. The program provides concrete examples of the concepts explained in the text assignment and by the experts who appear in the video.

As you watch the video program, consider the following questions:

1. How does Sheila Vaughn define adolescence?

2. According to Ellen Greenberger, what is involved in puberty—adolescent biological development?

3. What is the significance of the fact that physical development proceeds at a faster pace than intellectual and social development?

4. What are some of the concerns and problems occasioned by adolescent sexual development?

5. Why is it important to recognize teenagers' demand for independence as an aspect of normal development?

6. What do Greenberger and David Elkind say about why teenagers seem so egocentric and self-absorbed, and can be very self-conscious?

7. What are the principal features of adolescent intellectual development?

8. What, according to Joe White, are the positive and negative aspects of the fact that teenagers begin to develop a capacity for creative and advanced logical thinking?

9. What is the significance of adolescents' tendency to be in conflict and to rebel against authority?

10. What are the characteristics of adolescent moral development?

11. What are some of the ways teenagers show that they are developing awareness of social problems?

12. How do peer groups influence adolescent development?

13. Why do experts consider the idea that adolescence is characterized by turmoil a myth?

Review Exercises

Vocabulary Check

Match the following key terms and concepts with the appropriate definitions from the list below.

1. ___ adolescence (p. 523; video)

2. ___ authoritarian parents (p. 519)

3. ___ authoritative parents (p. 519)

4. ___ induction (p. 518)

5. ___ menarche (p. 524)

6. ___ moral emotions (p. 512)

7. ___ power-assertion methods (p. 518)

8. ___ puberty (p. 523; video)

9. ___ resilience (p. 538)

10. ___ stage theory of moral reasoning (pp. 510–512)

11. ___ turmoil theory of anguish and rebellion in adolescent development (p. 525; video)

a. the age at which a person becomes capable of sexual reproduction

b. the onset of menstruation

c. parents who exercise too much power and give too little nurturance

d. a characteristic of individuals who were able to bounce back to normality in adulthood despite traumatic experiences and growing up in neglectful or abusive circumstances in their early years

e. parents who know how and when to discipline their children

f. the view that adolescent anguish and rebellion are necessary and inevitable, the means by which teenagers separate themselves psychologically from their parents and form their own identities

g. Lawrence Kohlberg's concept describing moral development as being divided into three levels of two stages each

h. a method of child rearing in which the parent appeals to the child's own resources, abilities, sense of responsibility, and feelings for others in correcting the child's misbehavior

i. empathy, shame, and guilt

j. approaches to child rearing in which the parent relies on such methods as threats, physical punishment, depriving the child of privileges, and taking advantage of being bigger and more powerful than the child

k. the period of development between puberty (a biological event) and adulthood (a social event)

Other Key Terms and Concepts

moral development
  (pp. 505–512; video)

peer group (video)

permissive parents (p. 519)

secondary sex characteristics
  (p. 524)

Completion

Fill each blank with the most appropriate term from the list of answers below.

12. The _____ method of child rearing tends to produce children who have moral feelings and behave morally. Parents who employ _____ methods of child rearing tend to rely on threats and punishments.

13. Morality is a complex phenomenon involving _____, _____, _____, and _____.

14. According to Kohlberg's theory, until about the age of 10 or 11, most children function at a level of moral reasoning termed _____, which is characterized by obeying rules because one is ordered to and is afraid of punishment for failure to obey.

15. Many critics argue that Kohlberg's hierarchy of levels and stages actually reflects _____ ability and education, not moral judgment.

16. Children of alcoholics are at greater risk of such problems as _____, _____, and _____ than are children of nondisturbed parents.

17. At puberty, male hormones prompt the onset of _____ and the growth of the _____.

18. Evidence indicates that not all adolescents develop the ability for what Piaget called _____ or for complex moral reasoning.

19. Some of the factors that can hinder an adolescent's ability to deal with the transition to adulthood are _____, _____, and _____.

20. Psychologists are now studying the origins of children's _____, their ability to cope and become relatively normal adults despite childhoods marked by poverty and such traumatic experiences as parental divorce or having alcoholic or abusive parents.

anxiety and
    depression

behaving in
    considerate and
    responsible ways

cognitive ability to
    evaluate moral
    dilemmas

death of a close
    relative

drug abuse and
    delinquency

empathy for others

formal operational
    thought

induction

the inner voice of
    conscience

nocturnal emissions

parental divorce

power-assertion

preconventional
    morality

resilience

serious illness

social inadequacy

testes, scrotum, and
    penis

verbal

True-False

Read the following statements carefully and mark each true (T) or false (F).

21. ____ The induction method of child rearing may often require a parent to threaten to stop loving the child.

22. ____ Humanist psychologist Carl Rogers contended that parents who provide conditions of "psychological safety and freedom" will allow their children to develop their creative potential.

23. ____ When preschool children become best friends, they will probably stay best friends for years thereafter.

24. ____ Kohlberg developed his theory of the stages of moral reasoning by carefully observing the ways children and adults treat one another.

25. ____ In Kohlberg's system, everyone can expect to reach the highest level, known as postconventional or "principled" morality.

26. ____ Most people who were abused as children do not, as parents, abuse their own children.

27. ____ Puberty is a psychological event and adolescence is a biological event.

28. ____ Adolescents' intellectual development may be influenced by sociocultural factors and each person's individual temperament.

29. ____ Extreme turmoil and unhappiness are characteristic of most people's adolescent experience.

Short-Answer Questions

As a final review exercise, write brief answers to demonstrate that you are achieving the learning objectives of this lesson.

1. Describe and distinguish between the induction method of child rearing and power-assertion methods and discuss the possible effects of each on the child.

2. Briefly describe Kohlberg's theory of moral development and discuss several criticisms of his theory.

3. Discuss the effect of childhood experience on the adult and discuss the implications of cases in which adults have overcome difficult childhoods.

4. Describe changes produced by hormones during puberty.

5. Describe intellectual development during adolescence.

6. Identify several factors that may help or hinder adolescents' ability to deal with the transition to adulthood.

Self-Test

1. In the induction method of child rearing, parents do **NOT** appeal to the child's

    a. own resources.

    b. fear of losing their love.

    c. affection for others.

    d. sense of responsibility.

2. In power-assertion methods of child rearing, the parents' justification for orders, instructions, or requests boils down to expecting the child to comply because

    a. "it makes sense."

    b. "it's the right thing to do."

    c. "I say so."

    d. "you're a good kid."

3. Which of the following is **NOT** one of Kohlberg's levels of moral development?

    a. preconventional morality

    b. conventional morality

    c. postconventional morality

    d. transconventional morality

4. There has been heated debate over both Kohlberg's work and the ideas of Carol Gilligan because they implied there are differences in the ways _____ think about moral problems.

    a. men and women

    b. children and adults

    c. educated people and uneducated people

    d. Americans and Europeans

5. Kohlberg's theory of moral development has been criticized for
   a. reflecting verbal sophistication more than moral development.
   b. evaluating moral reasoning, not moral behavior.
   c. assuming that children are more moral than adults.
   d. ignoring the role of bias and prejudice.

6. The majority of the children of abusive or alcoholic parents
   a. acquire the problem of their parent.
   b. end up worse than their parent.
   c. grow up just fine.
   d. don't reach maturity.

7. Most children who are abused
   a. grow up to abuse their own children.
   b. do not, as parents, abuse their own children.
   c. never marry.
   d. marry, but never have children.

8. At puberty, the physical changes in boys are caused by hormones known as _____; the changes in girls, by hormones known as _____.
   a. androgens; estrogens
   b. estrogens; androgens
   c. epinephrine; norepinephrine
   d. endorphins; enkephalins

9. Which of the following adolescent problems is LEAST likely to be attributable to changes in hormone levels during puberty?
   a. feeling out of control of one's emotions
   b. being rebellious
   c. rapid mood swings
   d. growth spurts

10. There is _____ in the onset and length of puberty.
    a. little variation between boys and girls
    b. little individual variation
    c. enormous individual variation
    d. enormous sociocultural variation

11. During adolescence, most teenagers make the transition from Piaget's _____ stage to his _____ stage of cognitive development.
    a. sensorimotor; concrete operations
    b. concrete operations; formal operations
    c. preoperational; concrete operations
    d. sensorimotor; preoperational

12. Teenagers who are able to think abstractly and to reason deductively, using the premises common to their culture, have reached Piaget's _____ stage of cognitive development.
    a. sensorimotor
    b. preoperational
    c. concrete operations
    d. formal operations

13. According to research, which of the following does NOT seem to help those adolescents who have the fewest emotional upsets during the transitions to adulthood?
    a. supportive families
    b. good coping skills
    c. reliance on the positive evaluation of peers and parents
    d. a sense of purpose and self-confidence

14 . Which of the following is **NOT** true of the majority of teenagers' experience making the transition to adulthood?

    a.   They have supportive families.

    b.   They have a sense of purpose and self-confidence.

    c.   They have good friends and the skill to cope with problems.

    d.   They have suffered parental divorce, the death of a close relative, or serious illness.

Study Activities

The following activity challenges you to use your critical thinking and demonstrate how what you are learning can be applied to you and your own life. Try this activity and/or those your instructor assigns.

Many people who write novels and short stories do in a big way what this exercise is asking you to do on a much smaller scale. Re-create your teen years, go back to your past, and relive those exciting years of adolescence. The idea is to find, in memories of your own experiences—which, if they were at all typical, must have been vivid and memorable—examples of what you have been studying in this lesson. Even if you are still in your late teens, you will by now have gained some perspective on what you went through as a younger teen. If it's been many years since your adolescence, you probably have lasting recollections of that period in your life and should have strong opinions about teenagers, particularly if you have children of your own.

There are two good ways to approach this project systematically. You can organize your flashback chronologically, year by year, examining all the different things you remember during those periods. You can also think about aspects of your adolescence and describe each of them across your entire teen experience. Try both and decide which gives you the most confidence that you are fully and fairly revealing what you felt and thought in that period of transitions that, at the time, probably seemed impossible to understand.

As you describe what you remember about your teen self, first concentrate on your strong impressions of what seemed important then. As you start writing down some of these things and compare and evaluate them, you'll be able to decide if they were truly world-shaking crises or not. Be sure to record feelings; adolescence is a time of strong emotions and mood swings. Think about your great loves and hates, your triumphs and disasters. List all the physical changes you recall, when they occurred, what you thought about them, and how they seemed to compare with what was happening to your peers.

Indicate what and who gave you the most trouble. How did you get along at home, in school, in jobs? Did you have more trouble with the physical and social transitions from childhood to adolescence or from adolescence to adulthood? Explain your answer in terms of your thoughts, feelings, and recollections of your activities and accomplishments. Record what you liked most (what you miss) about your teen years, and what you disliked most.

Finally, after completing this activity, decide if today's teenagers are very much different from those of your time. Admittedly, there are different kinds of teenagers in each era, and you may have been wilder (or not wild at all) compared both to your contemporaries and to today's teens. In general, however, decide if adolescence today seems to be something unlike your teen experience. If you think so, indicate specific factors that may account for the difference you perceive.

Adulthood and Aging

Assignments

For the most systematic coverage of this lesson, we suggest that you complete the assignments in the sequence listed below.

Before viewing the video program:

- Read the "Learning Objectives" and "Overview" for this lesson. Use the Learning Objectives to guide your reading, viewing, and thinking.

- Read the "Viewing Notes" for this lesson.

- Read Chapter 14, "Development over the Life Span," pages 529–537, and Chapter 8, "Behavior in Social and Cultural Context," pages 274–275, in the Wade and Tavris text. First, familiarize yourself with their contents by reading the Chapter Outlines. As you read, note terms and concepts set in bold or italic type, especially those defined in the margins. Take the Quick Quizzes to check your understanding of material being described and explained.

View the video program, "Adult Development"

After viewing the video program:

- Briefly note your answers to the questions at the end of the "Viewing Notes."

- Review all reading assignments for this lesson, including the Summaries at the end of Chapters 14 and 8 in the textbook.

- Complete the "Review Exercises" to strengthen your understanding of this lesson's central concepts and terminology. Pay special attention to the "Vocabulary Check" exercise and the additional terms and concepts that follow—page references indicate where in the text assignment each term is defined. [Remember: there is a complete Glossary at the end of the text.]

- Take the "Self-Test" to measure the degree to which you are achieving this lesson's learning objectives. Check your answers against the "Answer Key" and review when necessary.

- Follow the suggestions in the "Study Activities" section at the end of this lesson and complete any other activities and projects assigned by your instructor.

Learning Objectives

When you have completed all assignments in this lesson, you should be able to:

1. Describe the general theories about aging and identify the contributions of research in gerontology.

2. Describe and evaluate the significance of menopause, midlife assessment, and the so-called midlife crisis.

3. Summarize the key features of Erik Erikson's theory of psychosocial development and analyze the differences between adult and child developmental stages.

4. Discuss how transition or milestone theorists view adult development, identify the principal kinds of transitions, and describe several major milestones in most people's lives.

5. Explain how circumstance and chance can influence adult development, and describe the roles of continuity and change in the adult experience.

6. Recognize the difference between transition and crisis, and develop guidelines for better planning.

Overview

Growing up doesn't mean development stops. Just because individuals get through childhood and adolescence doesn't mean they no longer face changes in what they do and what they are. This lesson shows that adult development, though not as rapid or dramatic as the earlier transformations, is nonetheless interesting and undeniably significant.

The lesson describes the general theories about aging, including the recent notion that aging is not natural and inevitable. It highlights the tremendous breakthroughs that have been achieved in the relatively new field of **gerontology**, the study of aging and the old.

Among the topics covered in this lesson are **menopause**, **midlife assessment**, and the so-called **midlife crisis**.

Erik Erikson's **theory of psychosocial development** is described in detail, and its many stages are delineated. Students are shown the differences between the stages of child development and those of adult development. The accuracy and utility of stage theories are analyzed.

The lesson discusses how chance and circumstance influence adult development. It is shown that both continuity and change play a role in adult development.

The work of transition or milestone theorists is presented. Principal transitions and milestones in people's lives are described, and **transitions** are distinguished from crises. Strategies for coping with transitions to prevent them from becoming crises are offered.

Viewing Notes

The video program entitled "Adult Development" supplements and amplifies the material covered in the video lessons on adolescent development and cognitive development. Together, the three programs provide a memorable introduction to the subject of human development and to the important theories about the changes individuals experience from conception to death. This program features the special problems and challenges of adult development.

As you watch the video program, consider the following questions:

1. What are the eight stages of Erikson's psychosocial theory of development, and what is the importance of that theory?

2. What does Judith Stevens-Long identify as the limitations of Erikson's theory?

3. How does Carl Broderick distinguish child development from adult development?

4. What do transition theories of development focus upon?

5. What sorts of problems are faced by young adults just starting out?

6. What factors does Broderick identify as contributing to successful and enjoyable parenthood?

7. What are some of the ways in which parenthood may affect people's self-perception, emotions, and feelings toward others—especially their own parents?

8. How does someone recognize if he or she is experiencing a midlife crisis?

9. What are some of the difficulties and rewards that adults who return to school can expect?

10. How do Jack Hansue's experiences with retirement validate Carol Humple's definition of the period of retirement as the "option years"?

11. Do all individuals who go through the same transitions experience them in the same way?

Review Exercises

Vocabulary Check

Match the following key terms and concepts with the appropriate definitions from the list below.

1. ___ generational identity (p. 275)

2. ___ gerontologists (p. 534)

3. ___ identity crisis (p. 530; video)

4. ___ menopause (p. 533)

5. ___ "midlife crisis" (p. 533; video)

6. ___ psychosocial theory of development (p. 530; video)

7. ___ "social clock" (pp. 532–533; video)

8. ___ stage theories (pp. 529–531; video)

9. ___ transitions (p. 532; video)

a. the cessation of menstruation; usually a gradual process lasting up to several years

b. Erik Erikson's theory that everyone passes through eight developmental stages

c. concepts holding that the physical and psychological development of children and adults involves passing through a number of phases or stages

d. what Erikson considered to be the major conflict of adolescence

e. a society's timetable for the "right" ages to marry, have children, start work, retire, and have other adult experiences

f. people who study aging and the old, whose research has challenged stereotypes and dramatically changed our understanding of old age by distinguishing processes that are part of normal aging from those due to preventable conditions

g. the ages of 16 to 24 seem to be especially critical for its formation

h. the controversial notion that people in their middle years go through an emotional crisis as they lament their lost youth and unfulfilled dreams

i. the changes from one role or situation to another; that is, events that happen (or fail to happen) that cause people and their lives to change in some way

Other Key Terms and Concepts

crisis (pp. 530–531)

crystallized intelligence
  (p. 535)

fluid intelligence (p. 535)

parenthood (p. 530; video)

retirement (video)

widows and widowers (video)

Completion

Fill each blank with the most appropriate term from the list of answers below.

10. The field of _____ has made astonishing advances in separating the processes that are normal in aging from those that are a result of illness or preventable conditions.

11. According to Erik Erikson's theory of _____, people pass through eight stages of development, and each stage represents a combination of _____ and _____.

12. Among the major milestones in life are _____, _____, and _____.

13. A factor that is fairly consistent throughout life is one's _____.

14. A _____ is a sudden, severely upsetting situation that forces you to mobilize your resources; a _____ is a change in your roles, routines, or relationships.

basic personality

biological drives

crisis

divorce

gerontology

getting married

having children

psychosocial development

societal demands

transition

True-False

Read the following statements carefully and mark each true (T) or false (F).

15. ____ Gerontology is one of the oldest scientific specialties.

16. ____ Most women go through menopause with no particular psychological difficulties and very few physical ones.

17. ____ Erik Erikson, a psychoanalyst, believed, as did Freud, that people are propelled principally by sexual motives.

18. ____ Both child development and adult development are powerfully governed by maturational and biological changes that are dictated by each person's genes.

19. ____ One's generational identity lasts throughout adulthood.

20. ____ All the people of roughly the same age who shared the experience of the Great Depression or the Vietnam War are likely to be influenced in their ideas and attitudes by the so-called cohort effect.

21. ____ Two ways to prevent a transition from becoming a crisis are to set reasonable expectations and not to be afraid to ask for help from friends, relatives, or support groups.

Short-Answer Questions

As a final review exercise, write brief answers to demonstrate that you are achieving the learning objectives of this lesson.

1. Describe the general theories about aging and identify the contributions of research in gerontology.

2. Describe and evaluate the significance of menopause, midlife assessment, and the so-called midlife crisis.

3. Summarize the key features of Erik Erikson's theory of psychosocial development and analyze the differences between adult and child developmental stages.

4. Discuss how transition or milestone theorists view adult development, identify the principal kinds of transitions, and describe several major milestones in most people's lives.

5. Explain how circumstance and chance can influence adult development, and describe the roles of continuity and change in the adult experience.

6. Recognize the difference between transition and crisis, and develop guidelines for better planning.

Self-Test

1. The two main theories of aging disagree principally on
   a. if there is a midlife crisis.
   b. if there is a male menopause.
   c. whether or not aging is natural and inevitable.
   d. whether or not aging is attributable to diet.

2. _____ is the scientific specialty that has made great strides in separating the processes that are normal in aging from those that result from illness or preventable conditions.
   a. Psychology
   b. Sociology
   c. Biology
   d. Gerontology

3. Menopause, the cessation of menstruation, is
   a. due to a deficiency disease.
   b. purely psychological.
   c. brought on when the ovaries stop producing estrogen and progesterone.
   d. reversible.

4. In a large survey of thousands of randomly chosen women, the majority characterized their experience of menopause as
   a. a medical crisis.
   b. a psychological crisis.
   c. something that goes largely unnoticed.
   d. positive or with no particular feelings at all.

5. From the example in the video, it is clear that, after midlife assessment, actions such as returning to college

    a. are bound to prove fruitless.

    b. can be enormously rewarding.

    c. are remarkably easy.

    d. are now characteristic choices for most older adults.

6. According to Erikson, each stage of development represents

    a. biological drives and societal demands.

    b. sexual motives and physiological capacities.

    c. a crisis.

    d. cultural standards and psychological desires.

7. Which of the following stages in Erikson's theory of development does **NOT** apply to adults?

    a. intimacy versus isolation

    b. trust versus mistrust

    c. generativity versus stagnation

    d. ego integrity versus despair

8. Because child development is more powerfully governed by maturational and biological changes dictated by the genes than is adult development, children tend to be _____ than middle-aged adults or old people.

    a. more emotional

    b. less predictable

    c. more alike

    d. less alike

9. What affects people the **LEAST** psychologically about transitions is

    a. whether or not they occur.

    b. whether the transition is expected or unexpected.

    c. the demand to change roles or take action.

    d. whether they are "on time" for their age.

10. Being fired from a job, the death of a spouse, and flunking out of school are examples of

    a. anticipated transitions.

    b. unanticipated transitions.

    c. nonevent transitions.

    d. chronic hassle transitions.

11. Adults tend to evaluate their development according to a _____ that determines if they are successfully meeting expectations about the progress of their lives.

    a. stage theory

    b. transition theory

    c. social clock

    d. climacteric

12. Each generation has its own identity, such as "Baby Boomers" or "Generation X," which lasts throughout adulthood; the critical period for the formation of a generational identity is

    a. later in life.

    b. from age sixteen to twenty-four.

    c. mid-life.

    d. puberty.

13. Circumstance (what people do and the conditions under which they work and live)

    a. cannot overcome biological motivation.

    b. can always be shaped by careful planning.

    c. is almost entirely dependent on chance.

    d. can challenge us to grow and mature.

14. People's best-laid plans and deepest aspirations are often kept from fulfillment by chance events and
    a. psychological problems.

    b. moral weaknesses.

    c. economic factors.

    d. the distraction of other options.

15. Among the several factors that can turn a transition into a crisis is
    a. having all your friends and family trying to help you deal with a change.

    b. facing a change that is unplanned and unanticipated.

    c. actually getting something you planned and worked for.

    d. having to concentrate on one problem to the exclusion of all others.

16. Which of the following is NOT one of the guidelines for preventing transitions from turning into crises?
    a. Avoid taking on too many life-shaking changes at once.

    b. Set reasonable expectations.

    c. Keep yourself constantly ready for unexpected stresses and crises.

    d. Ask for help when you need it.

17. Which of the following is NOT always a factor influencing how a person copes with the death of his or her spouse?
    a. the structure of routine and satisfying activities

    b. the cause of the deceased spouse's death

    c. how many friends and social connections the surviving spouse continues to have

    d. the financial resources of the surviving spouse

Study Activities

The following activity challenges you to use your critical thinking and demonstrate how what you are learning can be applied to you and your own life. Try this activity and/or those your instructor assigns.

Whatever your age, your life history has no doubt already included personal crises and transitions, and you will face many others in the future. From your study of this lesson, you should now appreciate that there are important differences between a transition and a crisis. The purpose of this exercise is to examine your own life experience to give you practice in identifying the differences between transitions and crises and to demonstrate your understanding of how to cope with such changes and events.

Make a list, or draw a timeline, starting with the date of your birth and extending into the foreseeable future. Write down all those events you consider major milestones in your development and note the progress of your various activities—in your physical and cognitive development, your education, your personal and family life, and your career. A timeline can be particularly revealing, since things stand out more clearly and relationships are clearer than on a list or in a narrative.

After you have completed your list or timeline, think about the entries you made. Which of the events or changes you included could be characterized as transitions and which as crises? Be sure you have, in fact, included all the real crises you've faced, not just successful or unavoidable changes and transitions. Once the crises are identified, ask yourself how you dealt with them. Had you prepared for them? Had you developed good enough coping skills to ease you through them? Did you have others to call on for assistance during the critical period? By systematically improving your knowledge of how you have dealt with crises in the past, you should improve your ability to deal with others in the future.

As to the future, extend your list or timeline into the coming years. Pencil in expected changes, events, and transitions you know are coming and should try to be ready for. Also indicate what unanticipated crises are possible, or even probable, and consider how they might be handled should they occur.

Health, Stress, and Coping

Assignments

For the most systematic coverage of this lesson, we suggest that you complete the assignments in the sequence listed below.

Before viewing the video program:

- Read the "Learning Objectives" and "Overview" for this lesson. Use the Learning Objectives to guide your reading, viewing, and thinking.

- Read the "Viewing Notes" for this lesson.

- Read Chapter 15, "Health, Stress, and Coping," in the Wade and Tavris text. First, familiarize yourself with its contents by reading the Chapter Outline. As you read, note terms and concepts set in bold or italic type, especially those defined in the margins. Take the Quick Quizzes to check your understanding of material being described and explained.

View the video program, "Health, Stress, and Coping"

After viewing the video program:

- Briefly note your answers to the questions at the end of the "Viewing Notes."

- Review all reading assignments for this lesson, including the Summary at the end of Chapter 15 in the textbook.

- Complete the "Review Exercises" to strengthen your understanding of this lesson's central concepts and terminology. Pay special attention to the "Vocabulary Check" exercise and the additional terms and concepts that follow—page references indicate where in the text assignment each term is defined. [Remember: there is a complete Glossary at the end of the text.]

- Take the "Self-Test" to measure the degree to which you are achieving this lesson's learning objectives. Check your answers against the "Answer Key" and review when necessary.

- Follow the suggestions in the "Study Activities" section at the end of this lesson and complete any other activities and projects assigned by your instructor.

Learning Objectives

When you have completed all assignments in this lesson, you should be able to:

1. Summarize Hans Selye's theory of the General Adaptation Syndrome.

2. Explain how a person's physical response to stress relates to his or her evaluation of the stressful event and ability to cope.

3. Explain the basic focus and assumption of the field of psychoneuroimmunology, and discuss the relationship between psychological processes and the immune system.

4. Describe several sources of stress (e.g., major life-change events, bereavement and tragedy, daily hassles, and continuing problems).

5. Define coping, describe the three general categories of coping with a problem, and discuss coping strategies relating to each category.

6. Describe various individual factors that can affect health and a person's ability to cope with stress.

7. Explain the concept of control and discuss several benefits and possible misuses.

8. Explain how social relationships can both help in coping and cause stress.

9. Discuss the controversy concerning the relationship between psychological factors and health and illness.

Overview

This lesson may come closer to each student's personal experience than any other. Not everyone is interested in the biology of behavior, the mechanisms of memory, or the stages of human development, but everyone has an idea about what stress is and knows it is important to be able to cope with it. This lesson defines stress, shows how it is related to physical illness, and suggests ways of coping.

Hans Selye's pioneering work, *The Stress of Life*, and his theory of the **General Adaptation Syndrome (GAS)** are covered in the text and the video program. It is explained how Selye worked out the relationship between physical and psychological stressors and people's experience of stress. The lesson discusses Selye's work on the interplay between stress and healthy adaptation to it and between stress and illnesses caused by it.

The lesson describes studies amplifying Selye's ideas, particularly with regard to how a person's physical responses to stress or evaluation of a stressful event may modify the stress and the person's capacity to cope. The fascinating field of **psychoneuroimmunology** is introduced, and the relationship between psychological processes and the immune system is explained.

Various sources of stress are described, **coping** is defined, and general categories of coping and coping strategies are explained. The lesson discusses individual factors that can influence one's health and ability to cope. It examines the positive and negative aspects of the concept of **locus of control** and reveals how social relationships can contribute to coping or can cause stress. The lesson also confronts the general issue of the mind-body connection, the controversy over the relationship between psychological factors and health and illness.

Viewing Notes

The video program "Health, Stress, and Coping" furnishes first-person testimony on coping with stress and dealing with stress-related illness. Among the people who appear in the program is Norman Cousins, who had successfully struggled against cancer, demonstrating to many that one's mind and spirit might play a role in helping the immune system fight disease.

Cousins and various experts discuss Hans Selye's General Adaptation Syndrome (GAS), the relationship between stress and physical illness, and various coping strategies for dealing with psychological stress.

As you watch the video program, consider the following questions:

1. What was Hans Selye's principal discovery?

2. How does Bernard Towers distinguish disease from "dis ease"?

3. How does Norman Cousins explain the connection between stress and illness?

4. How does Towers define psychoneuroimmunology?

5. What does Robert Lieberman say about posttraumatic stress disorder (PTSD)?

6. Why does Deborah Phillips characterize loss as a major source of stress?

7. What are some of the physical symptoms of stress?

8. What are some of the strategies for coping with stress offered in this program?

9. Why is it that some people seem to thrive in stressful situations, or seem to have a natural hardiness?

Review Exercises

Vocabulary Check

Match the following key terms and concepts with the appropriate definitions from the list below.

1. ___ coping (p. 560)

2. ___ emotion-focused coping (p. 562)

3. ___ General Adaptation Syndrome (GAS) (pp. 546–547; video)

4. ___ health psychology (p. 545)

5. ___ hostility (p. 553)

6. ___ locus of control (p. 557)

7. ___ posttraumatic stress disorder (PTSD) (video)

8. ___ primary control (p. 559)

9. ___ problem-focused coping (p. 562)

10. ___ psychological stress (p. 547; video)

11. ___ psychoneuroimmunology (PNI) (pp. 550–551; video)

12. ___ psychosomatic (p. 549)

13. ___ secondary control (p. 559)

14. ___ Type A personality (pp. 552–553)

a. the field that studies the relationships among psychology, the nervous system, and the immune system

b. an effort to accept external reality by changing one's own attitudes, goals, or emotions; a "learn to live with it" method of coping

c. according to Hans Selye, the bodily reactions to environmental stressors

d. the cynical or antagonistic attitude that can greatly increase the likelihood of getting coronary heart disease

e. a set of personal qualities that have been thought to increase the risk of heart attack (a conclusion that has become controversial)

f. a coping strategy that concentrates on changing or managing the emotions the problem has caused

g. cognitive and behavioral efforts to manage demands, in the environment or in oneself, that one feels are stressful

h. the result of a relationship between the person and the environment, in which the person believes the situation is overwhelming and threatening his or her well-being and ability to cope

i. a general expectation about whether the results of one's actions are under one's own control (internal locus) or beyond one's control (external locus)

j. a condition of chronic anxiety resulting from experience with danger or any serious trauma or stress and which is marked by periods of worry and irritability, depression, bad moods, and outbursts of hostility and aggression

k. a field within psychology that studies psychological aspects of health and illness

l. a coping strategy that attacks the problem itself

m. a term that describes the interaction between a physical illness or condition and psychological states

n. an effort to modify external reality by changing other people, the situation, or events; a "fighting-back" method of coping

Completion

Fill each blank with the most appropriate term from the list of answers below.

15. The General Adaptation Syndrome (GAS) is Hans Selye's description of the _____ reaction to _____.

16. Studies since Selye's work have found that stress is not a purely _____ condition that can lead directly to illness.

17. The basic assumption of _____ is that all disease is the result of relationships among the endocrine, nervous, and immune systems; behavior; and emotions.

18. The sources of stress include major life events, such as the _____, and smaller problems, the _____ that can wear us down over time.

19. The three general categories of coping are _____ the problem, _____ the problem, and _____ the problem but lessening the physical effects of its stress.

20. Personality factors may predispose individuals to certain diseases. For example, people who suppress their feelings almost all of the time have the personality trait of _____ and are at greater risk of becoming ill and even of dying sooner than people who can acknowledge their feelings of anxiety, anger, or fear.

21. What it is about Type A behavior that is dangerous to health: _____, not the irritability or anger that everyone feels on occasion, but the toxic kind that is cynical or antagonistic and characterizes people who are mistrustful of others and quick to have mean, furious arguments.

22. People with an _____ locus of control often deal more effectively with problems and decisions than people who lack this sense of mastery, who have an _____ locus of control.

23. Research has shown that for people with average, everyday levels of stress, social support had _____ on health; among people with above-average levels of stress, support from friends _____ their physical and emotional symptoms.

24. The connections that have been made between stress and illness have created a controversy over what some call the _____ of illness.

biological	helped reduce	psychoneuroimmunology
body's	hostility	rethinking
daily hassles	internal	solving
death of a loved one	learning to live with	stressors
emotional inhibition	no effect	
external	"psychologizing"	

True-False

Read the following statements carefully and mark each true (T) or false (F).

25. ____ Selye recognized that psychological factors, such as emotional conflict or grief, could be as important as physical factors, such as heat, toxic chemicals, and noise, in causing the General Adaptation Syndrome (GAS).

26. ____ Virtually all individuals behave about the same way when they are under stress.

27. ____ Psychoneuroimmunology has proved that stress affects the immune system, but there is no evidence that other systems—such as the cardiovascular, gastrointestinal, and endocrine—are similarly affected.

28. ____ Many researchers believe that most people are able to withstand acute (short-term) stress—even massive blows from major life events—but few people can cope forever with interminable, chronic stress.

29. ____ Relaxation and exercise are two methods that enable people to reduce stress as part of the coping strategy of living with a problem.

30. ____ Hard-driving workaholics are more prone to stress-related diseases and most invariably have heart attacks.

31. ____ In general, a sense of control is a good thing, but believing that an event or situation is controllable does not always lead to reduction in stress, and believing that an event or situation is uncontrollable does not always lead to an increase in stress.

32. ____ Friends can increase your stress as well as help you cope with it; as, for example, through the so-called contagion effect, by which, as you try to help them, their emotional problems "rub off" on you, making you depressed and troubled too.

33. ____ It is the goal of psychology to find ways to eliminate all stress and consequently all stress-related ailments.

Short-Answer Questions

As a final review exercise, write brief answers to demonstrate that you are achieving the learning objectives of this lesson.

1. Summarize Hans Selye's theory of the General Adaptation Syndrome.

2. Explain how a person's physical response to stress relates to his or her evaluation of the stressful event and ability to cope.

3. Explain the basic focus and assumption of the field of psychoneuroimmunology, and discuss the relationship between psychological processes and the immune system.

4. Describe several sources of stress (e.g., major life-change events, bereavement and tragedy, daily hassles, and continuing problems).

5. Define coping, describe the three general categories of coping with a problem, and discuss coping strategies relating to each category.

6. Describe various individual factors that can affect health and a person's ability to cope with stress.

7. Explain the concept of control and discuss several benefits and possible misuses.

8. Explain how social relationships can both help in coping and cause stress.

9. Discuss the controversy concerning the relationship between psychological factors and health and illness.

Self-Test

1. Which of the following is **NOT** one of the three phases of Selye's General Adaptation Syndrome?
   a. phase of intensification
   b. alarm phase
   c. phase of resistance
   d. phase of exhaustion

2. The important mediator between a stressor and the amount of stress it produces is
   a. the endocrine system.
   b. the immune system.
   c. the individual's evaluation of the stressor.
   d. a problem-solving strategy that is guaranteed to lead to a solution, if one exists.

3. Because people differ in how they interpret events and in how they respond to them, many psychologists now prefer a definition of stress, termed psychological stress, which is seen as the relationship between the _____ and the _____.
   a. stressor; stress
   b. stress; illness
   c. stress; individual
   d. individual; environment

4. Today's field of psychosomatic medicine recognizes that
   a. the mind controls the body.
   b. the body controls the mind.
   c. the mind and body affect each other.
   d. neither the mind nor the body affect the other.

5. In a study of medical students with the herpes virus, it was found that outbreaks were more likely to occur when the students were feeling loneliest or were under greatest stress, leading to the conclusion that

    a. people who are alone are more likely to suffer a herpes eruption.

    b. loneliness and stress suppressed their cells' immune capability.

    c. stress causes herpes.

    d. herpes is a psychosomatic disease.

6. Which of the following is NOT usually considered to be a powerful source of stress?

    a. spouse dying

    b. getting a divorce

    c. buying a new house

    d. continuing and uncontrollable daily hassles

7. What makes something a hassle is

    a. that fact that it is inherently unpleasant.

    b. your ability to handle it.

    c. what other people say about it.

    d. your feelings about it.

8. Which of the following is NOT one of the general strategies for coping with a problem?

    a. identifying the problem

    b. solving the problem

    c. rethinking the problem

    d. learning to live with the problem but lessening the physical effects of its stress

9. Which of the following is **NOT** one of the three goals of rethinking described by Shelley Taylor, who has worked with cancer and cardiac patients, women who have been raped, and other victims of disaster or disease?

   a. to find meaning in the experience

   b. to regain mastery over the event and one's life

   c. to keep the negative reality of what has happened from entering one's consciousness

   d. to restore self-esteem

10. Which of the following is **NOT** one of the possible factors that relates emotion to disease?

   a. emotional inhibition

   b. a positive, confronting emotional style

   c. a pessimistic attitude

   d. a sense of not having control

11. An important goal of health psychology is prevention, elimination of risk factors before illness develops; but among the obstacles to this is people's

   a. belief that illness, like death, is inevitable and unavoidable.

   b. insistence on waiting until they are so ill they must see a doctor.

   c. ignorance of the basic rules of how to protect their health.

   d. lack of incentive to change unhealthy habits.

12. A sense of control _____ the neuroendocrine and immune systems.

   a. has no discernible effects on

   b. directly affects

   c. is affected by but does not affect

   d. is nullified by the actions of

13. If an unrealistically confident person tries to control the uncontrollable, the resulting failure may lead to

    a.   an effort to find something controllable to deal with.

    b.   the self-deluding conclusion that someone or something else caused the failure.

    c.   helplessness in the face of uncontrollable stressful events.

    d.   renewed efforts based on a more realistic estimate of the chances for success.

14. Which of the following is NOT one of the ways in which friends can help you cope?

    a.   emotional support (providing concern and affection)

    b.   try to cheer you up, rather than let you talk about your problem

    c.   cognitive support (helping you evaluate problems and plan a course of action)

    d.   tangible support (offering resources and services)

15. What is probably the most important thing friends can do to help you cope with problems?

    a.   give you a feeling of attachment to others, of being part of a network that cares

    b.   give you money

    c.   offer advice

    d.   get you professional help, whether you want it or not

16. Regarding the long chain of connections between emotions and illness,

    a.   most researchers think that psychological factors count for nothing.

    b.   almost everyone agrees that health is largely mind over matter.

    c.   it is obvious that disease is a purely biological matter.

    d.   most researchers agree that these links should not be oversimplified.

17. A psychologically healthy person

   a. finds a way to solve all problems.

   b. relies on other people—friends, relatives, or professionals—to solve his or her problems.

   c. avoids problems whenever possible.

   d. faces problems, copes with them, and gets beyond them.

Study Activities

The following activity challenges you to use your critical thinking and demonstrate how what you are learning can be applied to you and your own life. Try this activity and/or those your instructor assigns.

One of the most intriguing aspects of the study of health, stress, and coping is the field known as psychoneuroimmunology. To engage in a study activity related to that subject, you would expect that a laboratory and years of scientific specialization might be required. Happily, this is not the case.

Read the section entitled "Emotional Inhibition" on pages 553–554 of the Wade and Tavris textbook. As this passage suggests, you may duplicate the research described. Over the coming weeks (or for as long as you wish to test the validity of the research on yourself), you can keep a diary like the ones mentioned. Just write down, as the impulse to do so strikes you, your "deepest thoughts and feelings" about anything and everything. If James Pennebaker's research is correct, this form of confession, this venting of inhibited emotions and thoughts, can provide physiological release and cognitive perspective that could reduce stress-related ailments to which you might be prone.

Be sure that you review the text passage thoroughly, to get the clearest possible idea of what you're trying to achieve. If the topic captures your interest, you may want to take the trouble to read the Pennebaker articles listed in the text's bibliography. Remember that the exercise may not be therapeutic if it becomes an obsession that may bring your deepest memories of traumatic events to the surface and, at the same time, make them more troublesome. Go systematically and carefully, doing only what the text passage and the articles indicate, and you may see some interesting, positive results.

Lesson 20

Psychological Disorders I

Assignments

For the most systematic coverage of this lesson, we suggest that you complete the assignments in the sequence listed below.

Before viewing the video program:

- Read the "Learning Objectives" and "Overview" for this lesson. Use the Learning Objectives to guide your reading, viewing, and thinking.

- Read the "Viewing Notes" for this lesson.

- Read Chapter 16, "Psychological Disorders," pages 575–594, in the Wade and Tavris text. First, familiarize yourself with its contents by reading the Chapter Outline. As you read, note terms and concepts set in bold or italic type, especially those defined in the margins. Take the Quick Quizzes to check your understanding of material being described and explained.

View the video program, "What Is Normal?"

After viewing the video program:

- Briefly note your answers to the questions at the end of the "Viewing Notes."

- Review all reading assignments for this lesson, including the Summary at the end of Chapter 16 in the textbook.

- Complete the "Review Exercises" to strengthen your understanding of this lesson's central concepts and terminology. Pay special attention to the "Vocabulary Check" exercise and the additional terms and concepts that follow—page references indicate where in the text assignment each term is defined. [Remember: there is a complete Glossary at the end of the text.]

- Take the "Self-Test" to measure the degree to which you are achieving this lesson's learning objectives. Check your answers against the "Answer Key" and review when necessary.

- Follow the suggestions in the "Study Activities" section at the end of this lesson and complete any other activities and projects assigned by your instructor.

Learning Objectives

When you have completed all assignments in this lesson, you should be able to:

1. Describe several differing definitions of abnormal behavior (psychological or mental disorder) and discuss some of the implications of the fact that mental health professionals do not always agree on what "normal" is.

2. Identify the primary function and purpose of the *Diagnostic and Statistical Manual of Mental Disorders*, and explore the controversy arising from such attempts to label and classify disorders.

3. Describe the symptoms of several anxiety disorders.

4. List and describe the various characteristics of mood disorders, including major depression and bipolar disorder.

5. Explore various theories about the origin of depression and why it seems to be more prevalent among females.

6. Identify and briefly describe the characteristics of the major personality disorders.

Overview

The heart of this lesson is the ongoing debate over the nature of **abnormality**; that is, over how to define mental or psychological disorder. Both the video and the text focus on the issue. The point is made that despite the fact that many people are being treated for psychological disorders characterized by abnormal behavior, experts can't agree on what "abnormal" means.

Another professional debate is described in this lesson. This one is over the classifications and diagnostic categories in the American Psychiatric Association's *Diagnostic and Statistical Manual of Mental Disorders*, which clinicians of all theoretical orientations use to diagnose psychological disorders of literally every kind. The text assignment includes revealing information on how the diagnostic categories for the *DSM* are selected. It shows that the process can be influenced by social and political factors as well as scientific considerations. Even publication of a much-expanded edition (*DSM-IV*) in 1994 did little to quiet the controversies engendered by that work's predecessors.

The lesson provides detailed descriptions of various **anxiety disorders** and their symptoms. It describes mood disorders, including **major depression** and **bipolar disorder**, and examines various theories on the origins of depression. The textbook emphasizes **vulnerability-stress models** which hold that depression (and many other psychological problems and mental disorders) result from an interaction between individual vulnerabilities—in personality traits, habits of thinking, genetic predisposition, and so forth—and environmental stress or sad events.

Major **personality disorders**, including **antisocial personality disorder**, are also discussed in this lesson.

Viewing Notes

The video program "What Is Normal?" helps in two ways to distinguish between normality and abnormality. First, it shows that some people with psychological disorders clearly have something wrong with them. Although their plight may be a "normal" thing, it is also a bad thing—an unpleasant thing few of us would want to experience. Second, the program lets leading authorities, researchers, and clinicians explain what they, in their daily work dealing with psychological disorders, have come to regard as the distinction between normal and abnormal. The program also shows why such working definitions continue to be debated.

The program also deals with the *Diagnostic and Statistical Manual of Mental Disorders (DSM)* and the controversy over its approach and its value.

As you watch the video program, consider the following questions:

1. Why is it so hard to define abnormal behavior, and how do the experts interviewed in the video program define it?

2. How does the *Diagnostic and Statistical Manual of Mental Disorders (DSM)* help psychologists and psychiatrists make objective diagnoses of abnormal behavior and psychological problems?

3. How is the *DSM* organized to classify various disorders?

4. What are some of the drawbacks and weaknesses of the *DSM* that its critics have cited?

5. What are the symptoms of depression, and why is it sometimes called the common cold of mental illness?

6. What has research identified as the most probable causes of depression?

7. What are some of the ways clinicians treat depression?

8. What is research such as that of Tony Strickland revealing about the biochemical nature of the relationship between stress and depression?

9. What are the characteristics of chronic anxiety and panic attacks?

10. What is thought to cause anxiety disorders?

11. How do clinicians treat panic attacks?

Review Exercises

Vocabulary Check

Match the following key terms and concepts with the appropriate definitions from the list below.

1. ___ abnormality (psychological or mental disorder) (pp. 576–577; video)

2. ___ agoraphobia (p. 584; video)

3. ___ antisocial personality disorder (p. 592)

4. ___ anxiety (pp. 581–582; video)

5. ___ bipolar (manic-depressive) disorder (p. 587)

6. ___ compulsions (p. 584)

7. ___ generalized anxiety disorder (p. 582)

8. ___ major depression (p. 586; video)

9. ___ narcissistic personality disorder (p. 592)

10. ___ obsessions (p. 584)

11. ___ panic attack (pp. 582–583; video)

12. ___ panic disorder (p. 582)

13. ___ paranoid personality disorder (p. 592)

14. ___ personality disorders (p. 592)

15. ___ phobia (p. 583)

a. a condition characterized by antisocial behavior, a lack of social emotions, and impulsivity

b. a continuous state of anxiety that occurs more days than not over a six-month period, marked by various physical symptoms but no physical cause

c. an adaptive, general state of apprehension that prepares an individual to cope with danger

d. repetitive, ritualized, stereotyped behavior that a person feels must be done to avoid disaster

e. any behavior or emotional state that causes personal suffering, that is self-destructive, or that is maladaptive and disrupts the person's relationships or the larger community

f. psychological disorders in which rigid, maladaptive personality patterns cause personal distress or an inability to get along with others

g. a brief feeling of intense fear and impending doom or death, accompanied by intense physiological symptoms, such as rapid breathing and pulse, sweaty palms, and dizziness

h. an unrealistic fear of a specific situation, activity, or object

i. "fear of fear"; a set of phobias, often set off by a panic attack, sharing the basic fear of being away from a safe place or person

j. a mood disorder involving disturbances in emotion (e.g., excessive sadness), behavior, cognition (e.g., low self-esteem), and body function

k. a disorder characterized by an exaggerated sense of self-importance and self-absorption

l. recurrent, unwished-for, persistent thoughts and images

m. a condition in which people worry about future panic attacks and regard each attack as a sign of impending death or disaster

n. unreasonable and excessive suspiciousness, jealousy, and mistrust

o. a mood disorder in which depression alternates with mania

Other Key Terms and Concepts

Diagnostic and Statistical Manual of Mental Disorders (DSM) (pp. 577–581; video)

normal hallucinations (p. 576)

obsessive-compulsive disorder (OCD) (p. 584)

posttraumatic stress disorder (PTSD) or acute stress disorder (p. 582)

vulnerability-stress models of mental disorders (pp. 588–589, 593–594)

Completion

Fill each blank with the most appropriate term from the list of answers below.

16. Definitions of "abnormal" depend on who is doing the defining. Among the definitions of abnormal behavior are _____, _____, _____, and _____.

17. The primary aim of each edition of the *Diagnostic and Statistical Manual of Mental Disorders* has been _____: to provide clinicians and researchers of all theoretical orientations with clear criteria for diagnostic categories.

18. Generalized anxiety disorder may show such symptoms as _____, _____, _____, and _____.

19. Bipolar disorder is also known as _____ disorder.

20. Biological theories account for the origin of depression in terms of _____ and/or _____.

21. Two common personality disorders are the _____ personality and the _____ personality.

22. People who have antisocial personalities have problems in behavioral inhibition and lack two critical emotions: _____ and guilt.

brain chemistry	genetic factors	paranoid
descriptive	irritability	restlessness
difficulty concentrating	maladaptive behavior	sleep disruption
emotional distress	manic-depressive	statistical deviation
empathy	narcissistic	violation of cultural standards

True-False

Read the following statements carefully and mark each true (T) or false (F).

23. ____ After years of wrangling, psychologists have finally agreed on a single working definition of abnormality.

24. ____ The *DSM-IV* severely reduced the number of mental disorders it describes.

25. ____ Panic attacks are part of a genuine psychological disorder but are self-actuated by people who want attention and sympathy.

26. ____ People with obsessions and compulsions are suffering from forms of anxiety disorder.

27. ____ Depression is so widespread, it has been called "the common cold of mental illness."

28. ____ PET scans, which show changes in the metabolism of glucose in the brain, provide graphic evidence of the fact that the brain of a person with bipolar disorder operates differently when the person is experiencing depression than when he or she is undergoing a manic episode.

29. ____ People with antisocial personalities include mass murderers (serial killers), swindlers, and some people whose political and economic success may be attributable to their antisocial attitudes.

Short-Answer Questions

As a final review exercise, write brief answers to demonstrate that you are achieving the learning objectives of this lesson.

1. Describe several differing definitions of abnormal behavior (psychological or mental disorder) and discuss some of the implications of the fact that mental health professionals do not always agree on what "normal" is.

2. Identify the primary function and purpose of the *Diagnostic and Statistical Manual of Mental Disorders*, and explore the controversy arising from such attempts to label and classify disorders.

3. Describe the symptoms of several anxiety disorders.

4. List and describe the various characteristics of mood disorders, including major depression and bipolar disorder.

5. Explore various theories about the origin of depression and why it seems to be more prevalent among females.

6. Identify and briefly describe the characteristics of the major personality disorders.

Self-Test

1. One of the main reasons psychologists and other experts, not to mention laypersons, can't agree on a definition of abnormality is that
   a. they refuse to grant that anyone is sufficiently knowledgeable to put forth such a definition.
   b. the people in one field don't acknowledge the validity or utility of definitions made by people in another field.
   c. they can't agree on a definition of what is normal.
   d. new kinds of abnormality keep appearing all the time.

2. The authors of the text choose to define mental disorder as
   a. any behavior or characteristic that sets a person apart from the others in his or her community.
   b. acting or being obviously different.
   c. being emotionally disturbed or mentally unbalanced.
   d. any behavior or emotional state that causes an individual great suffering or worry, that is self-defeating or self-destructive, or that is maladaptive and disrupts the person's relationships or the larger community.

3. The *Diagnostic and Statistical Manual of Mental Disorders* is prepared and published by
   a. the American Psychological Association.
   b. the American Psychiatric Association.
   c. *Psychology Today* magazine.
   d. the Surgeon General of the United States.

4. Some critics of the *Diagnostic and Statistical Manual of Mental Disorders* are seriously concerned that
   a. a diagnosis can create a self-fulfilling prophecy.
   b. the *DSM* does not include enough categories of disorder.
   c. a person's medical or physical history is thought to be irrelevant to a psychiatric diagnosis.
   d. women and children are grouped together in many diagnostic categories.

5. In addition to diagnostic categories, the *Diagnostic and Statistical Manual of Mental Disorders* classifies disorders according to five _____, or clinically important factors.

   a. measures

   b. indices

   c. areas

   d. axes

6. Generalized anxiety disorder is marked by

   a. a sudden onset of symptoms.

   b. continuous anxiety that has occurred more days than not in a six-month period.

   c. fear of being away from a safe place or person.

   d. delusions of grandeur.

7. There are many _____, or unrealistic fears of a specific situation, activity, or thing.

   a. compulsions

   b. obsessions

   c. phobias

   d. manias

8. A man who feels he must wash his hands and face eight times before leaving the house, and a woman who cannot begin a meal unless each piece of china and each utensil is in exactly the same spot as at the start of all previous meals, are suffering from

   a. phobias.

   b. compulsions.

   c. obsessions.

   d. mania.

9. Which of the following is **NOT** among the symptoms experienced in major depression?

    a.   exaggerated sense of self-importance

    b.   loss of appetite or overeating

    c.   trouble concentrating

    d.   loss of sexual desire

10. _____ of the people who go through a bout of major depression will do so only once.

    a.   Nearly all

    b.   Only a few

    c.   About half

    d.   None

11. Feeling _____ is characteristic of someone in the manic phase of bipolar disorder.

    a.   hopeless and without direction

    b.   full of ambitions, plans, and power

    c.   fearful and withdrawn

    d.   anxious

12. Which of the following is **NOT** among the most common theories of the origins of depression?

    a.   biological theories

    b.   social theories

    c.   attachment theories

    d.   bipolar theories

13. One reason more women than men seem to suffer from episodes of major depression is that

    a. there is evidence that women are genetically predisposed to depressive disorders.

    b. women's place in society is depressing.

    c. men are more likely to engage in behavior, such as drug use and violence, that masks the symptoms of depression.

    d. men avoid acting depressed precisely because depression is a "women's disease."

14. Which of the following is NOT characteristic of a personality disorder?

    a. It is related to an episode of illness or depression.

    b. It involves rigid, maladaptive, consistent traits that cause great personal distress.

    c. It involves an inability to get along with others.

    d. It is a repeated, long-term pattern of behavior.

15. A person who exhibits pervasive, unfounded suspiciousness and mistrust of other people, irrational jealousy, expectations of trickery, secretiveness, and doubt about the loyalty of others is probably suffering from

    a. posttraumatic stress disorder.

    b. paranoia.

    c. obsessive-compulsive disorder.

    d. multiple personality disorder.

16. Ronald has been diagnosed as having an antisocial personality. One day he is arrested in the act of robbing a convenience store. At the police station, he appears truly sorry for what he has done and says the money was needed to help his sick mother. It is likely that he

    a. is feeling intensely emotional.

    b. is lying.

    c. feels remorse but cannot control his behavior.

    d. was misdiagnosed, because antisocial personalities may think about committing crimes but do not carry out their fantasies.

Study Activities

The following activity challenges you to use your critical thinking and demonstrate how what you are learning can be applied to you and your own life. Try this activity and/or those your instructor assigns.

Now that you've learned that even the experts haven't been able to agree on a definition of abnormality or abnormal behavior, you can get into the act. Since there are so many definitions being used and abused, it can't really hurt for you to try to define the concept too. It may even help you understand the subject by forcing you to focus on all that must be accounted for in the notions of "normal" and "abnormal."

Before you ever thought of taking this course, you must have had some idea of what was abnormal. As children we start building a working vocabulary of terms that describe various degrees of abnormality: crazy, insane, mad, demented, nuts, wacko, strange, weird, zany, out of your mind, off your head, sick, bonkers, addled, balmy, lunatic, loony, schizo, bizarre, kooky, eccentric, off the wall, way out, bent—the list can go on endlessly. This should be a hint that either many people seem to be different or many people think about what is normal and what isn't—or both. There's something funny and a bit frightening about a world in which experts can't decide what abnormal means but everyone seems to go around sticking labels that say "abnormal" on people.

In this exercise, try to be more serious than just trying to pick the best label. Your goal should be to get the clearest picture in your own mind of what it means to be abnormal. For example, you might encounter homeless people who behave in ways that appear far from normal. Decide what it is about such people that should be called abnormal. Do they talk to themselves uncontrollably? Do they move in jerky, almost mechanical fashion, or remain conscious but motionless for long periods? Do they talk or act violently? Do they engage in ritual behavior, doing or saying the same things over and over again? Do people you know who are not homeless former mental patients fit any of the foregoing descriptions? Do people you know act strangely when drinking or using drugs? Would you call them normal or abnormal?

Are retarded people or autistic people abnormal? Are disabled people or people whose appearance—height, weight, hair length—varies from the average abnormal? Are skinheads abnormal? Were hippies abnormal? What about people with unconventional political or religious ideas? Is it possible there is no such thing as abnormality, but merely an almost-infinite set of variations on the normal theme—a continuum on which some people are farther apart, farther out, than others? You get the point. Pursue this analysis on your own by observing people's behavior and fitting them into your list of normal or abnormal types. Try to concentrate on behavior, not just people. You should be evaluating what people do more than who or what they are. Don't forget your own behavior. What do you do that someone else might consider abnormal?

Lesson 21

Psychological Disorders II

Assignments

For the most systematic coverage of this lesson, we suggest that you complete the assignments in the sequence listed below.

Before viewing the video program:

- Read the "Learning Objectives" and "Overview" for this lesson. Use the Learning Objectives to guide your reading, viewing, and thinking.

- Read the "Viewing Notes" for this lesson.

- Read Chapter 16, "Psychological Disorders," pages 578, 595–611, in the Wade and Tavris text. First, familiarize yourself with its contents by reading the Chapter Outline. As you read, note terms and concepts set in bold or italic type, especially those defined in the margins. Take the Quick Quizzes to check your understanding of material being described and explained.

View the video program, "Psychotic Disorders"

After viewing the video program:

- Briefly note your answers to the questions at the end of the "Viewing Notes."

- Review all reading assignments for this lesson, including the Summary at the end of Chapter 16 in the textbook.

- Complete the "Review Exercises" to strengthen your understanding of this lesson's central concepts and terminology. Pay special attention to the "Vocabulary Check" exercise and the additional terms and concepts that follow—page references indicate where in the text assignment each term is defined. [Remember: there is a complete Glossary at the end of the text.]

- Take the "Self-Test" to measure the degree to which you are achieving this lesson's learning objectives. Check your answers against the "Answer Key" and review when necessary.

- Follow the suggestions in the "Study Activities" section at the end of this lesson and complete any other activities and projects assigned by your instructor.

Learning Objectives

When you have completed all assignments in this lesson, you should be able to:

1. Discuss the various aspects of dissociative disorders and examine the controversial nature of dissociative identity disorder (multiple personality disorder [MPD]).

2. List and briefly describe the various somatoform disorders.

3. List the *DSM-IV* criteria for substance abuse and explain the basic tenets of the biological or disease model and the learning model of addiction.

4. List and briefly describe the more common symptoms of schizophrenia, and distinguish schizophrenia from multiple personality disorder.

5. Describe important features of the prevalent theories about the causes of schizophrenia.

6. List and describe several categories of organic brain disorders that can produce psychotic symptoms.

7. Identify the myths and danger signs of suicide.

Overview

This second lesson on psychological disorders deals with several fascinating, even famous, mental problems. **Dissociative disorders** are examined, including **amnesia** and **dissociative identity disorder** (**multiple personality disorder**, popularized in books and films such as *The Three Faces of Eve* and *Sybil*), and amnesia. The lesson also describes **somatoform disorders**, apparently medical problems manifesting physical symptoms but with no demonstrable medical cause.

Addiction and the use and abuse of alcohol and other drugs is discussed. The **biological or disease model of addiction** and the **learning model of addiction** are described in detail and compared.

Schizophrenia is extensively discussed; its symptoms are described, and it is distinguished from multiple personality disorder, with which laypersons often confuse it. It is carefully explained that schizophrenia is not just one disorder but, rather, an umbrella term that encompasses a number of severe disorders that may differ in kinds of symptoms, duration, and severity. The challenging issue of the causes of schizophrenia is presented, including accounts of some recent research on the genetic aspects of the disorder. There is also coverage of recent research on the possibility that brain abnormalities —including those caused by prenatal brain damage—may increase the likelihood of schizophrenia (as well as other mental disorders).

Organic brain disorders, which can have psychotic symptoms though they are caused by such factors as brain injuries, brain tumors, and poisoning, are described and compared to such disorders as schizophrenia, which they may resemble.

There is discussion of what each of us can do to help prevent friends from trying to commit suicide. The myths are revealed and the danger signs listed.

Viewing Notes

The video program "Psychotic Disorders" explores the severest of mental disorders. It shows what it is like to have a psychological disturbance such as schizophrenia and describes how such an illness can disrupt the lives of patients, friends, and families. Several experts evaluate the prospects for improving treatment and for finding the causes of these devastating ailments. The program examines the suspected causes of schizophrenia and discusses innovative approaches to successful treatment.

As you watch the video program, consider the following questions:

1. What do psychologists mean by "psychotic disorders"?

2. What are some of the different types of symptoms individuals with schizophrenia display?

3. What do PET scans reveal about the brains of people suffering from schizophrenia?

4. What evidence is there of a hereditary component to schizophrenia?

5. What evidence is there that stress plays a role in the development of schizophrenia?

6. What does research suggest about how schizophrenics process information?

7. What are some of the treatment approaches for schizophrenia?

Review Exercises

Vocabulary Check

Match the following key terms and concepts with the appropriate definitions from the list below.

1. ___ amnesia (p. 595)

2. ___ biological or disease model of addiction (pp. 599–600)

3. ___ conversion disorder (p. 578)

4. ___ dissociative disorders (p. 595)

5. ___ dissociative identity disorder (multiple personality disorder [MPD]) (p. 596)

6. ___ hypochondria (p. 578)

7. ___ learning model of addiction (pp. 601–603)

8. ___ psychosis (p. 605; video)

9. ___ schizophrenia (pp. 605–610; video)

10. ___ somatoform disorders (p. 578)

11. ___ substance abuse (p. 599)

12. ___ "word salads" (p. 606)

a. a psychotic disorder marked by some or all of these symptoms: delusions, hallucinations, incoherent word associations, inappropriate emotions, or lack of emotions

b. theory that regards addiction to alcohol or to any other drug as a biochemical process

c. extreme preoccupation with one's health and an unrealistic fear of disease

d. conditions under which normally integrated consciousness or identity is split or altered, as in psychogenic amnesia or multiple personality

e. a rare dissociative disorder marked by the appearance within one person of two or more distinct personalities, each with its own name, history, and traits

f. incoherent, loose word associations, symptomatic of schizophrenia

g. physical complaints that may last for several years with no demonstrable medical cause and with symptoms that are inconsistent with known physical diseases

h. theory holding that drug abuse and addiction reflect an interaction of physiology and psychology, of person, culture, and learning

i. partial or complete loss of memory for information or past events; when no organic causes are present, it is classified as a dissociative disorder

j. a single physical disturbance that seems to serve a psychological function, such as expressing a psychological conflict or need

k. any mental condition that involves distorted perceptions of reality, irrational behavior, and an inability to function in most aspects of life

l. a maladaptive pattern of substance use leading to clinically significant impairment or distress

Other Key Terms and Concepts

fugue state (p. 596)

organic brain disorders (video)

vulnerability-stress model of schizophrenia (p. 610)

Completion

Fill each blank with the most appropriate term from the list of answers below.

13. The most common dissociative disorder is _____, involving partial or complete loss of past memories; when no causes for this are apparent, this condition is referred to as _____.

14. The central characters in *Sybil* and *The Three Faces of Eve* suffered from _____.

15. Among the _____ disorders, which are characterized by physical symptoms with no demonstrable medical cause, are _____ and _____.

16. The *DSM-IV* distinguishes substance _____ from substance _____.

17. In the _____ model of addiction, the individual acquires a _____ for the drug.

18. Individuals who hear voices, feel invisible creatures crawling over them, laugh at sad news, and "know" that Martians can hear their thoughts are probably afflicted with _____.

19. Psychiatrist Donald Klein says that if depression is the common cold of psychiatry, schizophrenia is its _____.

20. Almost every expert studying schizophrenia believes it is a _____ disease.

21. Brain injuries, diseases, infections, nutritional deficiencies, and poisoning can cause _____ that can produce the symptoms of psychosis.

22. To be in a better position to prevent a suicide, you should be able to separate the myths from the facts about suicide, knowing, for example, that there are no _____ and that you must _____.

abuse	dissociative identity disorder (multiple personality disorder)	somatoform
amnesia		"suicidal types"
brain	hypochondria	take all suicide threats seriously
cancer	organic brain disorders	
conversion disorder	psychogenic	tolerance
disease	schizophrenia	use

True-False

Read the following statements carefully and mark each true (T) or false (F).

23. ____ Some experts think dissociative identity disorder (multiple personality disorder) is extremely rare and may even be concocted by psychiatrists and psychologists; others believe it isn't so rare but rather is often misdiagnosed as schizophrenia.

24. ____ Even though it is true that hypochondriacs sometimes get sick, just like anyone else, they do have an unrealistic fear of disease that seems to express a psychological need or conflict.

25. ____ According to the biological or disease model of addiction, people who have an addiction to drugs or alcohol can spread it to others through contagion.

26. ____ Opponents of the disease model of addiction note that not all addicts go through physiological withdrawal symptoms when they stop taking the drug.

27. ____ Schizophrenia is not the same as multiple personality; schizophrenia describes a fragmented condition—an impairment of the brain characterized by the inability to process emotions and cognitions as do people with "normal" brains—not the coexistence of several different personalities.

28. ____ Because of the contradictory findings of research into the causes of schizophrenia, some scientists believe that prevalent theories are actually describing several different disorders with different causes.

29. ___ There is now undeniable evidence that schizophrenia is caused by a virus.

30. ___ Brain tumors can cause psychotic symptoms only in people who are already predisposed to psychosis.

31. ___ If you are afraid a friend is in danger of committing suicide, don't risk making things worse by asking him or her: "Are you thinking of suicide?"

32. ___ If a friend is talking about suicide, that means he or she probably won't do it.

Short-Answer Questions

As a final review exercise, write brief answers to demonstrate that you are achieving the learning objectives of this lesson.

1. Discuss the various aspects of dissociative disorders and examine the controversial nature of dissociative identity disorder (multiple personality disorder [MPD]).

2. List and briefly describe the various somatoform disorders.

3. List the *DSM-IV* criteria for substance abuse and explain the basic tenets of the biological or disease model and the learning model of addiction.

4. List and briefly describe the more common symptoms of schizophrenia, and distinguish schizophrenia from multiple personality disorder.

5. Describe important features of the prevalent theories about the causes of schizophrenia.

6. List and describe several categories of organic brain disorders that can produce psychotic symptoms.

7. Identify the myths and danger signs of suicide.

Self-Test

1. Like posttraumatic stress disorder, dissociative disorders are often responses to
   a. genetic programming.
   b. faulty learning.
   c. a shocking event or series of events.
   d. chronic disease.

2. A person in a(n) _____ not only forgets his or her identity but also gives up customary habits and wanders far from home, perhaps even taking a new identity, remarrying, and getting a new job.
   a. addictive state
   b. altered state of consciousness
   c. state of amnesia
   d. fugue state

3. Which of the following is a form of somatoform disorder?
   a. schizophrenia
   b. multiple personality disorder
   c. organic brain disorder
   d. conversion disorder

4. Someone who complains of physical symptoms without demonstrable medical cause probably is subject to
   a. hypochondria.
   b. somatoform disorder.
   c. obsessive-compulsive disorder.
   d. conversion disorder.

5. In diagnosing somatoform disorders, clinicians look for symptoms

    a. of organic disease.

    b. that are inconsistent with known physical diseases or with basic anatomy and for which no organic cause can be found.

    c. of malingering.

    d. of multiple personality.

6. Which of the following is **NOT** one of the several *DSM-IV* symptoms of abuse of alcohol or any other drug?

    a. failure to fulfill role obligations

    b. regular, moderate use that has gone on for many years

    c. persistent conflicts with other people about use of substance or cause by the substance

    d. use of the substance in hazardous situations

7. The biological or disease model of addiction

    a. has been largely replaced by the learning model.

    b. is widely accepted by researchers and the public.

    c. is accepted by few researchers.

    d   applies only to individuals with genetic predispositions to substance abuse and addiction.

8. In the learning model, drug addiction or abuse is **MOST** likely to be found in people

    a. who believe they are stronger than the drug.

    b. whose social customs teach occasional, moderate use of the drug.

    c. who use the drug as a means of coping with problems or stress.

    d. who avoid frequent use and potent forms of the drug.

9. Schizophrenics are **LEAST** likely to manifest

    a. bizarre delusions.

    b. auditory, visual, or tactile hallucinations.

    c. a heightened ability to get along with other people.

    d. severe emotional abnormalities.

10. The severity, duration, and symptoms of schizophrenia
    a. depend on the age of the sufferer.

    b. vary.

    c. are much the same for all schizophrenics.

    d. are not the same for men as for women.

11. Because schizophrenic thought is often an illogical jumble of ideas and symbols, linked by meaningless rhyming words or by remote associations, the incoherent speech of severe schizophrenics has been termed
    a. glossolalia.

    b. run-on sentences.

    c. poetic.

    d. word salads.

12. Regarding the prognosis for people with schizophrenia, psychiatrists often speak of the _____: of all people diagnosed and hospitalized with schizophrenia, one-third will recover completely, one-third will improve significantly, and one-third will not get well.
    a. dementia dimensions

    b. praecox probability

    c. rule of thirds

    d. role of chance

13. Which of the following is NOT one of the theories of the causes of schizophrenia?
    a. family or other pressures

    b. biological theories

    c. the vulnerability-stress model

    d. the humanistic-cognitive model

14. A possible breakthrough in identifying the origins of schizophrenia is growing evidence that _____ factors and _____ may be at work.

    a. cultural; the environment

    b. genetic; brain abnormalities

    c. situational; parental influence

    d. unknown; forces

15. Syphilis, if it goes untreated, can lead to _____, a deterioration in mental and motor functioning that ends in paralysis, psychosis, and death.

    a. dementia praecox

    b. Huntington's chorea

    c. paresis

    d. gonorrhea

16. Although they both may have the same symptoms, unlike some schizophrenics, someone with an organic brain disorder, such as brain damage or a brain tumor, would not be able to _____ on occasion.

    a. interrupt his or her "madness," to seemingly turn off the symptoms

    b. respond to treatment

    c. be released from institutionalized care

    d. escape into unresponsive withdrawal

17. It is one of the danger signs of a depressed person being at risk of trying to commit suicide when he or she

    a. falls deeper and deeper into depression.

    b. reveals specific plans for carrying out the suicide.

    c. never has tried to commit suicide before.

    d. talks about such things as how the suicide will hurt his or her family or break religious rules.

18. When you have strong reason to believe a friend may try to commit suicide, the most important thing to remember is

    a. don't do anything, because whatever you do might embarrass your friend.

    b. don't upset your friend by bringing in health professionals or calling a suicide hot line.

    c. don't leave your friend alone.

    d. it is better to do nothing than the wrong thing.

Study Activities

The following activity challenges you to use your critical thinking and demonstrate how what you are learning can be applied to you and your own life. Try this activity and/or those your instructor assigns.

Gain some in-depth knowledge of psychological disorders by doing some research and reading. Choose as your topic one of the disorders covered in this lesson. You'll probably learn more about the topic and researching such a topic if you focus on as narrow a subject as possible. You'll never learn all there is to know about schizophrenia, dissociative disorders, or substance abuse in general, but you might find it very interesting and enlightening to try to find out what amnesia or a fugue state is all about.

This is one of the occasions where outside reading is imperative. Your text and the video lessons are great introductions to psychology as a whole and to many specialized topics, but this exercise requires more than an introduction. You want to get more detail, more examples, and more points of view. The text's bibliography is a starting point; the library is even better. A major library would be the best—a library with back issues of psychological and psychiatric journals containing articles on all the subjects you've been learning about. In this regard, since this is an introductory course, no one expects you to start reading professional journals cover to cover. You can obtain considerable information from such periodicals without having to get a Ph.D. or M.D. first. Many books and magazines written for laypersons have articles on subjects you may want to investigate.

You'll know you've done enough reading on your chosen topic when you start telling other people about it and when you find yourself answering questions that arise in your reading before the book or article answers them. When this knowledge acquisition is well under way, start planning a report on what you've learned. Organize it around your original interest, explaining what you've learned and what misconceptions you've corrected. Try to be as thorough as necessary to supply all the fundamental facts that you would like to have had presented to you in one accessible paper when you started this project.

Lesson 22

Approaches to Therapy I

Assignments

For the most systematic coverage of this lesson, we suggest that you complete the assignments in the sequence listed below.

Before viewing the video program:

- Read the "Learning Objectives" and "Overview" for this lesson. Use the Learning Objectives to guide your reading, viewing, and thinking.

- Read the "Viewing Notes" for this lesson.

- Read Chapter 17, "Approaches to Treatment and Therapy," pages 617–629 and 646, in the Wade and Tavris text. First, familiarize yourself with its contents by reading the Chapter Outline. As you read, note terms and concepts set in bold or italic type, especially those defined in the margins. Take the Quick Quizzes to check your understanding of material being described and explained.

View the video program, "Approaches to Therapy"

After viewing the video program:

- Briefly note your answers to the questions at the end of the "Viewing Notes."

- Review all reading assignments for this lesson, including the Summary at the end of Chapter 17 in the textbook.

- Complete the "Review Exercises" to strengthen your understanding of this lesson's central concepts and terminology. Pay special attention to the "Vocabulary Check" exercise and the additional terms and concepts that follow—page references indicate where in the text assignment each term is defined. [Remember: there is a complete Glossary at the end of the text.]

- Take the "Self-Test" to measure the degree to which you are achieving this lesson's learning objectives. Check your answers against the "Answer Key" and review when necessary.

- Follow the suggestions in the "Study Activities" section at the end of this lesson and complete any other activities and projects assigned by your instructor.

Learning Objectives

When you have completed all assignments in this lesson, you should be able to:

1. Outline and briefly describe the three basic approaches to the treatment of psychological disorders.

2. Briefly review the history of the interrelationship between the medical (organic) model and the psychological (mental) model.

3. List and briefly describe the common types of drugs used to treat psychological disorders, and discuss the need for caution in the use of such medication.

4. Describe the use of psychosurgery and electroconvulsive therapy to help seriously disturbed people.

5. Briefly explain the basic principles of the psychodynamic ("depth" or "insight") therapies.

6. Briefly explain the basic principles of the cognitive and behavioral therapies.

7. Briefly explain the basic principles of the humanist and existential therapies.

8. Discuss some of the factors involved in knowing when to start or stop therapy and in choosing a therapist.

Overview

This lesson introduces the three basic approaches to the treatment of psychological disorders: **medical treatments, psychotherapy**, and **self-help and community alternatives**. The first two are described in detail in this lesson; the third is treated in the next lesson. The history of the medical (organic) model and the psychological (mental) model of treatment and their interrelationship are discussed.

The lesson describes drugs most commonly used to treat emotional problems and psychoses, including antipsychotic drugs, **antidepressants**, and **tranquilizers**. Their significant uses, actions, and side effects are discussed. The controversy over the use of **psychosurgery** and **electroconvulsive therapy (ECT)** is examined.

The basic principles of **psychodynamic ("depth" or "insight") therapies**, such as psychoanalysis, are explained, as are the ideas behind the **cognitive and behavioral therapies**, the **humanist and existential therapies**, and **eclectic** approaches. The video program and text assignment help distinguish one approach from the other by providing virtual side-by-side comparisons.

A separate section is devoted to identifying the factors that can help you become a smart therapy consumer.

Viewing Notes

The "Approaches to Therapy" video program features Hal, a man who is not mentally ill, but merely has an ordinary problem in living for which he seeks help through psychotherapy. Viewers observe therapeutic sessions with three different therapists, each of whom employs a different psychotherapeutic approach. Hal is shown interacting with the therapists, and viewers can see how the therapists apply different methods and concepts to the same problem. The therapists tell viewers about the techniques they use and explain that they may draw upon various therapeutic perspectives to employ a more eclectic approach.

As you watch the video program, consider the following questions:

1. What are the significant differences between the three forms of psychotherapy depicted in the video program?

2. How does Susan Brown describe psychoanalytic psychotherapy and her approach to using it to aid someone such as Hal?

3. How does Steven Sultanoff define and employ humanist, client-centered therapy?

4. What does Christine Padesky expect of herself in doing cognitive therapy with clients such as Hal, and what were her goals in the initial session with Hal, which appears in the program?

5. According to the three therapists featured in the video lesson, what is the value of combining various techniques in an eclectic approach to psychological problems?

6. What ideas do the therapists in the video program have about how clients can select the right therapist?

Review Exercises

Vocabulary Check

Match the following key terms and concepts with the appropriate definitions from the list below.

1. ___ antidepressant drugs (p. 619)

2. ___ antipsychotic drugs (major tranquilizers) (p. 619)

3. ___ aversive conditioning (pp. 625–626)

4. ___ behavioral therapies (pp. 625–627)

5. ___ client-centered (nondirective) therapy (p. 628)

6. ___ cognitive therapy (p. 627; video)

7. ___ electroconvulsive therapy (ECT) (p. 622)

8. ___ free association (p. 624)

9. ___ humanist therapies (p. 628; video)

10. ___ psychodynamic therapies (pp. 624–625; video)

11. ___ psychosurgery (p. 622)

12. ___ rational emotive behavior therapy (p. 627)

13. ___ systematic densensitization (pp. 625–626)

a. tranquilizers primarily used in the treatment of schizophrenia and other disorders involving psychotic symptoms, such as delusions

b. therapy that aims to change the disoriented or irrational thoughts involved in emotional problems and self-defeating actions

c. in psychoanalysis, a method of revealing unconscious conflicts by saying whatever comes to mind

d. "insight" or "depth" therapies, including orthodox Freudian psychoanalysis and its modern variations, which explore unconscious dynamics

e. drugs, such as stimulants, that influence neurotransmitters in the brain; usually used to treat mood and anxiety disorders

f. surgical procedures that destroy or isolate selected areas of the brain believed to be involved in emotional disorders or violent, impulsive behavior

g. a humanist therapy developed by Carl Rogers

h. the use of punishment to replace the positive reinforcement that perpetuates a bad habit

i. one of the earliest and best-known forms of cognitive therapy, developed by Albert Ellis

j. a step-by-step process of "desensitizing" a client to a feared object or experience

k. therapies that aim to help people feel better about themselves and reach "self-actualization"

l. a procedure occasionally used for cases of prolonged major depression, in which a brief brain seizure is induced to alter brain chemistry

m. therapies based on learning principles

Other Key Terms and Concepts

brief psychodynamic therapy (p. 625)

existential therapy (p. 629)

exposure treatment (flooding) (p. 626)

lobotomy (p. 622)

selective serotonin reuptake inhibitors (SSRIs) (p. 619)

therapeutic window (p. 621)

tranquilizers (p. 619)

transference (p. 624)

Completion

Fill each blank with the most appropriate term from the list of answers below.

14. The three basic approaches to treating psychological disorders are _____, _____, and _____.

15. For centuries, diagnoses and treatments of psychological disorders have alternately reflected either the _____ (organic) model or the _____ (mental) model.

16. A major breakthrough in the treatment of schizophrenia was achieved with the introduction of _____, such as chlorpromazine (Thorazine).

17. The challenge of using drugs to treat psychological disorders is to find the _____, the amount of any given drug that is enough to help but not so much that it can produce harmful side effects.

18. Critics argue that _____ is unreliable, produces unpredictable results, and can cause brain damage; supporters may counter with the contention that because some people are so out of control and are a constant danger to themselves and others, such drastic intervention is called for. Because of the legal and ethical problems involved, it is regarded as a procedure of last resort and is rarely used today.

19. The goal of psychodynamic therapies, such as _____, is _____, the patient's moment of truth, the awareness of the reason for his or her symptoms and anguish.

20. Therapists who practice cognitive or behavioral therapy aim to change a person's current _____ or _____.

21. Among the techniques used in behavioral therapy are _____, _____, _____, and _____.

22. A principal aim of _____, or nondirective, therapy is to build the client's self-esteem and help him or her self-actualize.

23. One of the most important factors in becoming a smart therapy consumer is _____.

antipsychotic drugs (major tranquilizers)

attitudes

aversive conditioning

behavior

client-centered

contracts

fees

flooding

insight

medical

medical treatments

psychoanalysis

psychological

psychosurgery

psychotherapy

self-help and community alternatives

systematic desensitization

"therapeutic window"

True-False

Read the following statements carefully and mark each true (T) or false (F).

24. ___ The medical treatment of emotional disorders and psychoses has largely been abandoned in favor of psychotherapy.

25. ___ Compared to the psychological model of mental disorders, the medical model is a relatively new approach.

26. ___ Tranquilizers seem to have little or no effect on depression, and people who use such drugs develop problems with withdrawal and tolerance.

27. ___ Within a given culture, men and women may not metabolize antidepressants and other drugs the same way.

28. ___ The proper use of drugs to treat emotional disturbances and psychoses depends on the individual, the problem, whether or not the physician is up-to-date on which drugs alleviate which problems and on the potential side effects of each drug, and on the drugs being combined with other therapy.

29. ___ Electroconvulsive therapy (ECT) is universally condemned and no longer used by reputable therapists.

30. ___ In psychoanalysis, patients have achieved transference when they get their parents or some other third party to pay the therapist.

31. ___ The behavioral technique known as systematic desensitization has been particularly effective in overcoming phobias, such as fear of flying.

32. ___ Research using PET scans shows changes in the brain function of individuals with obsessive-compulsive disorder before and after treatment with behavior therapy.

33. ___ Humanist therapists can only accept as clients self-actualized persons.

34. ___ In general, if you have a persistent problem that you don't know how to solve, one that causes you considerable unhappiness and that has lasted for six months or more, it may be time to look for help.

Short-Answer Questions

As a final review exercise, write brief answers to demonstrate that you are achieving the learning objectives of this lesson.

1. Outline and briefly describe the three basic approaches to the treatment of psychological disorders.

2. Briefly review the history of the interrelationship between the medical (organic) model and the psychological (mental) model.

3. List and briefly describe the common types of drugs used to treat psychological disorders, and discuss the need for caution in the use of such medication.

4. Describe the use of psychosurgery and electroconvulsive therapy to help seriously disturbed people.

5. Briefly explain the basic principles of the psychodynamic ("depth" or "insight") therapies.

6. Briefly explain the basic principles of the cognitive and behavioral therapies.

7. Briefly explain the basic principles of the humanist and existential therapies.

8. Discuss some of the factors involved in knowing when to start or stop therapy and in choosing a therapist.

Self-Test

1. The three basic approaches to the treatment of psychological disorders are
   a. humanistic, behavioral, and cognitive.
   b. psychotherapy, medical treatments, and self-help and community alternatives.
   c. drugs, psychosurgery, and electroconvulsive therapy (ECT).
   d. client-centered, therapist-centered, and problem-centered.

2. The emphasis in psychiatry in the late twentieth century has shifted from psychotherapy because of the evidence that some disorders have a genetic, _____, or neurological abnormality.
   a. mental
   b. biochemical
   c. brain
   d. emotional

3. Many experts contend that there is a _____ basis to many, and perhaps most, emotional disorders and psychoses.
   a. self-induced
   b. cultural
   c. humanistic
   d. biological

4. Tranquilizers are usually prescribed for people
   a. with schizophrenia and other psychoses.
   b. unable to sleep.
   c. who are nervous, anxious, and unhappy.
   d. with depressed mood, panic, or anxiety.

5. The most effective long-term treatment for people who suffer from a mood disorder with manic episodes is
   a. major tranquilizers.

   b. minor tranquilizers.

   c. antidepressants.

   d. lithium carbonate.

6. One study of the doses of antipsychotic drugs needed for optimal treatment showed that Asian schizophrenics required _____ Caucasian schizophrenics.
   a. exactly the same dosage as

   b. as much as ten times the dosage given to

   c. as little as one-tenth the dosage given to

   d. none of the drugs given to

7. Tricyclic antidepressants, such as _____, prevent the normal reabsorption, or "reuptake," of norepinephrine and serotonin by the cells that have released them. Selective seratonin reuptake inhibitors (SSRIs), such as _____, work on the same principle as the tricyclics but specifically target serotonin, boosting its levels.
   a. Thorazine; Stelazine

   b. Elavil; Prozac

   c. Valium; Xanax

   d. Lithium; Librium

8. Psychosurgery (such as lobotomies)
   a. has been entirely replaced by the use of antipsychotic drugs.

   b. is as widely practiced as ever.

   c. has been replaced by more refined operations that pinpo specific areas of the brain thought to be involved in er disorders and disturbed behavior, but is rarely used f

   d. has been banned by law.

9. Which of the following is **NOT** true of electroconvulsive therapy (ECT), so-called shock therapy?
    a.   may temporarily help people with prolonged major depression
    b.   is effective with many disorders, including schizophrenia and alcoholism
    c.   produces memory loss and other cognitive impairments
    d.   affects every aspect of brain activity

10. In orthodox psychoanalysis, patients usually meet with the analyst
    a.   once a week.
    b.   several times a week.
    c.   only in groups.
    d.   only in a hospital setting.

11. In brief psychodynamic therapy,
    a.   the therapist chooses a dynamic focus or central issue for the therapy.
    b.   treatment is limited to a year of three to five sessions per week.
    c.   the client reveals his or her entire history.
    d.   the main goal is to achieve insight into the client's unconscious and catharsis (release) from his or her symptoms and problems.

12. A behavior therapist would be **MOST** likely to help someone who wants to break a habit such as nail biting by use of
    a.   systematic densensitization.
    b.   aversive conditioning.
    c.   self-actualization.
    d.   a variable-ratio (VR) schedule of reinforcement.

13. The aim of cognitive therapy is to correct
    a.   improper conditioning through reconditioning.
    b.   inappropriate behavior by teaching people how to live with their fantasies.
    c.   biological imbalances caused by genetic errors.
    d.   distorted and unrealistic thinking.

14. The current relationship between cognitive and behavioral therapies is that
    a. behavioral therapies borrow from cognitive therapies.
    b. cognitive therapies borrow from behavioral therapies.
    c. behavioral therapies and cognitive therapies borrow from each other.
    d. behavioral therapies and cognitive therapies borrow from most other forms of psychotherapy.

15. Humanistic therapy concentrates on
    a. the here and now.
    b. the roots of problems in past situations, relationships, and behavior.
    c. the why and how, the reasons and causes of emotional problems.
    d. replacing bad habits with good ones.

16. Which of the following is **NOT** considered a form of humanistic therapy?
    a. Gestalt therapy
    b. behavior modification
    c. existential therapy
    d. client-centered (nondirective) therapy

17. Existential therapists believe that your life is not inevitably determined by your past or your circumstances, but, instead, that
    a. you can be conditioned to cope with adversity and be happy and productive.
    b. you have the power to choose your own destiny.
    c. proper medication and biological treatments should be used to shape your life.
    d. long-term analysis can reveal how to overcome past influences that may now be controlling your life.

18. All else being equal, it is most important for your therapist or counselor to be someone

    a.   who is a wise and empathic person.

    b.   who comes highly recommended.

    c.   who has one or more advanced degrees.

    d.   is licensed to do therapy.

19. Which of the following is **NOT** a good reason to consider ending therapy or changing therapists?

    a.   Therapy has become the most important thing in your life.

    b.   The therapist keeps finding new reasons for you to stay, though your original problems were solved long ago.

    c.   Your therapist has been unable to help you cope with the problems that brought you there.

    d.   You really expected a quick fix for your problem.

Study Activities

The following activity challenges you to use your critical thinking and demonstrate how what you are learning can be applied to you and your own life. Try this activity and/or those your instructor assigns.

If you have a psychological problem that is serious enough to require professional intervention, turn now to the section of the Wade and Tavris text called "Becoming a Smart Consumer of Therapy" (pages 646–647). That should get you started toward finding the right sort of help in dealing with what is troubling you. If you are no more unhappy, anxious, guilty, distracted, or otherwise emotionally out of sorts than most of the people around you, the following exercise may be both entertaining and instructive.

Consider the depiction of psychological disorders in art and popular culture. Survey all the movies, books, plays, television and radio programs, paintings, or other fine arts or popular arts for instances in which psychotherapy, psychiatry, mental hospitals, shock therapy, psychosurgery, drug therapy, or anything else to do with emotional and mental problems is portrayed.

No two people will compile the same information for this project. It all depends on what movies you've seen and what books you've read. You are not expected to go out and find examples of artistic depictions of madness or television shows featuring psychiatrists. You are expected to try remembering all the examples you can. The point is that mental illness and its treatment is an important theme in art and literature. Certain stereotypes have developed, and many misconceptions have been perpetuated. All of these contribute to the way we all think about mental health, mental illness, and the ways in which one is maintained and the other treated.

This exercise can be a great deal of fun, and quite easy. Just start with some obvious examples. Think about all the mad scientists, such as Dr. Frankenstein, in fiction and film. Think about all the characters in literature who are mad or go mad, including Shakespeare's Lady Macbeth and Ophelia. What about entire plays or films about the inmates of insane asylums or mental hospitals? *One Flew over the Cuckoo's Nest* comes to mind. There are fictionalized depictions of therapists, as in movies about psychiatrists or about Freud himself.

As you jot down your examples, decide if what was portrayed bore any relation to what you've learned about real mental problems and real therapy. Try to identify misleading stereotypes, unrealistic settings, characterizations, and explanations. The better you are able to tell what is invented or sensationalized from what is real, the better you will be able to understand and deal with real feelings, fears, ideas, and behavior. Incidentally, you may become a more perceptive critic of artistic creations.

Approaches to Therapy II

Assignments

For the most systematic coverage of this lesson, we suggest that you complete the assignments in the sequence listed below.

Before viewing the video program:

- Read the "Learning Objectives" and "Overview" for this lesson. Use the Learning Objectives to guide your reading, viewing, and thinking.

- Read the "Viewing Notes" for this lesson.

- Read Chapter 17, "Approaches to Treatment and Therapy," pages 625–646, in the Wade and Tavris text. First, familiarize yourself with its contents by reading the Chapter Outline. As you read, note terms and concepts set in bold or italic type, especially those defined in the margins. Take the Quick Quizzes to check your understanding of material being described and explained.

View the video program, "Therapy Choices"

After viewing the video program:

- Briefly note your answers to the questions at the end of the "Viewing Notes."

- Review all reading assignments for this lesson, including the Summary at the end of Chapter 17 in the textbook.

- Complete the "Review Exercises" to strengthen your understanding of this lesson's central concepts and terminology. Pay special attention to the "Vocabulary Check" exercise and the additional terms and concepts that follow—page references indicate where in the text assignment each term is defined. [Remember: there is a complete Glossary at the end of the text.]

- Take the "Self-Test" to measure the degree to which you are achieving this lesson's learning objectives. Check your answers against the "Answer Key" and review when necessary.

- Follow the suggestions in the "Study Activities" section at the end of this lesson and complete any other activities and projects assigned by your instructor.

Learning Objectives

When you have completed all assignments in this lesson, you should be able to:

1. Briefly explain the basic principles of family and group therapies.

2. Briefly describe some of the alternatives to traditional individual psychotherapy.

3. Summarize some of the problems involved with commitment of individuals with severe psychological disorders.

4. Discuss the efforts to evaluate the effectiveness of psychotherapy and its alternatives, and identify some of the factors involved in successful therapy.

5. Explore which therapies are most effective for certain problems.

6. Describe situations in which therapy might prove harmful.

7. Discuss three myths dealing with the value of therapy.

Overview

This lesson is a continuation of the discussion of therapy begun in Lesson 22. Here the emphasis is on alternatives to traditional individual, one-on-one therapies. The text and video lesson examine **family therapy**, **group therapy**, and **self-help** approaches. There are also evaluations of the effectiveness of various kinds of therapy and consideration of factors that contribute to successful therapy.

Some negative aspects of therapy are dealt with as well. The lesson addresses problems involved in commitment of severely disturbed individuals to institutions and the related problems that have arisen with the movement to deinstitutionalize such persons.

There is also discussion of situations in which therapy may prove harmful and of central myths that create dissatisfaction with therapy.

Among the positive information provided is data on the growing impact of **community programs** and **self-help support groups**, including such successful approaches as **rehabilitation psychology**.

Viewing Notes

The video program "Therapy Choices" continues the coverage of therapy started in the previous video lesson, "Approaches to Therapy." The program for this lesson focuses on alternatives to traditional individual psychotherapy. Three kinds of therapy are featured: family therapy, group therapy, and self-help approaches.

As you watch the video program, consider the following questions:

1. What roles do the therapist and the group participants play in group therapy?

2. Why do family therapists deal with the whole family instead of the individual?

3. What are the advantages and limitations of group therapy?

4. What are the advantages and limitations of family therapy?

5. What are the advantages and limitations of self-help approaches to problems?

6. How do each of the therapies in the program differ from one-on-one therapies?

Review Exercises

Vocabulary Check

Match the following key terms and concepts with the appropriate definitions from the list below.

1. ___ clubhouse model (p. 643)

2. ___ community programs (pp. 642–643)

3. ___ family therapy (pp. 629–631)

4. ___ rehabilitation psychology (p. 643)

5. ___ scientist-practitioner gap (pp. 633–634)

6. ___ self-help and support groups (pp. 644–645; video)

7. ___ therapeutic alliance (p. 636)

a. the bond of confidence and mutual understanding between therapist and client that allows them to work together to solve the client's problems

b. therapeutic and support programs intended to help people who are seriously mentally ill or who have chronic disabilities and need more than individual therapy

c. a field of psychology concerned with the assessment and treatment of people who are physically or mentally disabled, either temporarily or permanently

d. the breach between scientists and therapists on the issue of the relevance and importance of research findings; over the view that research is often irrelevant to therapy; that psychotherapy is an art, not a science; and that laboratory research and survey studies capture only a small and shadowy image of the real person

e. groups of individuals who face a similar problem and meet together to exchange information and provide mutual support

f. a form of therapy that views individual problems as existing within a family network

g. a program for mentally ill people that provides rehabilitation counseling, job and skills training, and a support network

Other Key Terms and Concepts

controlled clinical trials (p. 635)

empirically validated treatment (p. 638)

encounter groups (video)

genogram (p. 630)

group therapy (pp. 631–632)

Completion

Fill each blank with the most appropriate term from the list of answers below.

8. Some _____ therapists use a multigenerational approach, helping clients identify patterns of behavior that have been repeated across generations of their family.

9. Alternatives to traditional therapy include _____ and _____.

10. With self-help group members outnumbering _____ patients four to one, we are in something of a _____.

11. The policy of releasing disturbed people from institutions has been caused, in part, by the demands of the _____ and _____ movements.

12. _____ therapies are as diverse as their leaders, and in these therapies, ideally, members learn that their problems and fantasies are not unique.

13. Among the ways in which a client can be harmed by therapy are _____ of the client's emotional state and worsening of symptoms and _____ on the part of the client, who becomes unable to leave therapy and relies excessively on the therapist for all decisions.

14. Psychotherapist Bernie Zilbergeld contends that psychotherapy itself promotes central _____ that increase dissatisfaction with it.

civil-rights

community programs

dependency

deterioration

family

group

myths

patients'-rights

self-help and support groups

self-help revolution

therapy

True-False

Read the following statements carefully and mark each true (T) or false (F).

15. ____ Family therapy is particularly suited to children and adolescents with emotional or behavioral problems.

16. ____ Group therapies are commonly used in institutions and are popular among people who have a range of social difficulties, such as shyness and anxiety.

17. ____ Rehabilitation therapists work only with schizophrenics.

18. ____ Fortunately, most deinstitutionalized mental patients who stop taking their antipsychotic medication do not have their psychotic symptoms return.

19. ____ Most people who go through *any* therapy or self-improvement program will tell you they are the better for it.

20. ____ Good therapeutic candidates—successful patients or clients—combine a basically strong sense of self with sufficient distress to motivate them to change.

21. ____ Insight therapists are the most effective in dealing with depression.

22. ____ The effectiveness of psychotherapy depends to a great degree on the motivation of the clients.

23. ____ In his book, *The Shrinking of America*, Bernie Zilbergeld, himself a psychotherapist, argues that Americans are too attached to psychotherapy, and for the wrong reasons.

Short-Answer Questions

As a final review exercise, write brief answers to demonstrate that you are achieving the learning objectives of this lesson.

1. Briefly explain the basic principles of family and group therapies.

2. Briefly describe some of the alternatives to traditional individual psychotherapy.

3. Summarize some of the problems involved with commitment of individuals with severe psychological disorders.

4. Discuss the efforts to evaluate the effectiveness of psychotherapy and its alternatives, and identify some of the factors involved in successful therapy.

5. Explore which therapies are most effective for certain problems.

6. Describe situations in which therapy might prove harmful.

7. Discuss three myths dealing with the value of therapy.

Self-Test

1. The _____ perspective recognizes that if one family member is to benefit from therapy that produces change, the others must change too.

   a. humanistic

   b. family kaleidoscope

   c. family systems

   d. cognitive

2. In group therapy, ideally, members learn

   a. how to become more like other members of the group.

   b. how to keep from revealing their problems and innermost selves.

   c. that their problems and fantasies are not unique.

   d. where to find a good therapist.

3. The basic assumption underlying family therapy is that

   a. each family has strong members and weak members.

   b. all illnesses are due to the relationships that develop between parents and children.

   c. therapy is most effective if each member of the family is treated separately.

   d. an individual's problems arise in and must be solved in a family context.

4. People with mental retardation, epilepsy, chronic pain, severe physical injuries, cancer, addiction, and psychiatric problems are just some of the sorts of people who receive assessment and treatment from

   a. encounter groups.

   b. insight therapists.

   c. rehabilitation psychologists.

   d. psychometric psychologists.

5. Which of the following would be LEAST likely to be part of a self-help support group?

   a. women who have had mastectomies

   b. relatives of people with Alzheimer's disease

   c. abusive parents

   d. people with serious psychological disorders.

6. Community mental health centers

   a. tend to be inadequately funded to provide sufficient inpatient and outpatient services for released mental patients and others with psychological disorders.

   b. are ineffectual because of staff disagreements over which forms of therapy to employ.

   c. are probably an unconstitutional violation of patients' right to refuse treatment.

   d. have all but overcome the problems of deinstitutionalization and are getting most psychotic homeless people off the streets.

7. One of the more sensible solutions proposed to deal with the dilemma of mental patients who in prior years may have been institutionalized is

   a. massive reinstitutionalization.

   b. outpatient services.

   c. legal requirements that released patients stay on antipsychotic medication.

   d. making doctors and therapists responsible for the behavior and the welfare of deinstitutionalized individuals.

8. Economic pressures and the use of managed-care health programs are forcing psychotherapists to do all of the following EXCEPT

   a. justify what they do.

   b. produce clear guidelines for which therapies are effective.

   c. decide which therapies are best for which disorders.

   d. recommend self-help books to more and more of their clients.

9. Based on hundreds of studies, it appears that psychotherapy
   a. only works for people with enough money to pursue it for years.
   b. is better than doing nothing at all.
   c. works best with institutionalized patients.
   d. doesn't work at all.

10. Therapeutic effectiveness
    a. requires years of training and practice to achieve.
    b. is usually found only among practitioners whose fees are relatively high.
    c. depends on the bond between therapist and client called the therapeutic alliance.
    d. is seldom appreciated by their confused and troubled clients.

11. Tom and Jeff are therapist and client. They don't like each other, they are not at all alike, the come from different cultures, and they absolutely do not understand each other. How successful is Jeff's therapy likely to be?
    a. Its success will depend on the form of therapy that Tom practices.
    b. Its success will depend on how good a therapist Tom is.
    c. It is likely to be highly successful.
    d. It is not likely to be at all successful.

12. _____ relies on techniques derived from learning principles, not worrying about the client's past or unconscious anxieties.
    a. Psychoanalysis
    b. Behavior therapy
    c. Client-centered therapy
    d. Involuntary therapy

13. "Depth" therapies seem best suited to treating people who are

    a.   suffering from anxiety, fear, or phobias.

    b.   introspective about their motives and feelings and want to explore their pasts and understand why they are the way they are.

    c.   afflicted with severe personality problems.

    d.   sex offenders or have sex-related problems.

14. _____ has had its greatest success in the treatment of mood disorders, notably depression.

    a.   Psychoanalysis

    b.   Cognitive therapy

    c.   Client-centered therapy

    d.   Behavior therapy

15. Which of the following is **NOT** one of the ways it is thought a person in therapy can be harmed?

    a.   Therapist-induced disorders: the therapist consciously or unconsciously induces the client to produce symptoms of a problem the therapist zealously believes is prevalent.

    b.   Coercion: taking advantage of the therapeutic relationship to exert undue influence, including engaging in such unethical behavior as sexual intimacies and getting the client to behave in reprehensible ways.

    c.   Bias: the therapist not understanding the client because of the client's race, religion, sexual orientation, or ethnic group.

    d.   Rejection: the client refusing to follow the therapist's recommendations and seeking other therapeutic relationships.

16. A therapist strongly believes that the emotional problems of adult females typically stem from childhood sexual abuse. In treatment sessions, the therapist constantly encourages the client to look for such signs of abuse in her recollections of childhood. Eventually, the woman is convinced she remembers being raped by an uncle. This may be an example of

    a. an archetype.

    b. age repression.

    c. directive therapy.

    d. a pseudomemory.

17. Which of the following is **NOT** one of the three central myths that Bernie Zilbergeld believes are promoted by therapy and cause dissatisfaction with it?

    a. People should try to change because they are not as happy, as good, or as competent as they should be.

    b. Almost any change is possible; if something is wrong, fix it.

    c. Therapy will release the real you that's been locked inside you.

    d. Change is relatively easy.

18. Perhaps the greatest myth about therapy is that it can

    a. help you make decisions.

    b. transform you into someone you're not.

    c. make it easier to get through bad times when no one seems to care or understand.

    d. improve your morale and make it easier to cope.

Study Activities

These activities challenge you to use your critical thinking and demonstrate how what you are learning can be applied to you and your own life. Choose those activities that interest you most and/or those your instructor assigns.

1. Learn to be a smart therapy consumer. Review the section on this subject on pages 646–647 of the Wade and Tavris textbook. Look at the list (on page 632 in the textbook) of specific therapies best suited to particular problems. You may not need or want therapy right now, but the guidelines provided by the authors, both of whom are psychologists, could prove invaluable at some later time—for you or someone you care about.

2. Increase your awareness of the myths and stereotypes associated with therapy. You may want to consult Bernie Zilbergeld's *The Shrinking of America* to get some basic ideas and some suggestions on other sources of information.

3. Interview your closest friends and relatives concerning any particularly good or bad experiences they've had with psychotherapy. Find out what type of therapy they received, and what was positive or negative in their experience. Try to get them to be as specific as possible. Guide your inquiry by thinking about what you learned in this lesson. Don't forget to chronicle your own psychotherapeutic experiences.

Social Psychology

Assignments

For the most systematic coverage of this lesson, we suggest that you complete the assignments in the sequence listed below.

Before viewing the video program:

- Read the "Learning Objectives" and "Overview" for this lesson. Use the Learning Objectives to guide your reading, viewing, and thinking.

- Read the "Viewing Notes" for this lesson.

- Read Chapter 8, "Behavior in Social and Cultural Context," pages 263–278, 288–301, in the Wade and Tavris text. First, familiarize yourself with its contents by reading the Chapter Outline. As you read, note terms and concepts set in bold or italic type, especially those defined in the margins. Take the Quick Quizzes to check your understanding of material being described and explained.

View the video program, "Social Psychology"

After viewing the video program:

- Briefly note your answers to the questions at the end of the "Viewing Notes."

- Review all reading assignments for this lesson, including the Summary at the end of Chapter 8 in the textbook.

- Complete the "Review Exercises" to strengthen your understanding of this lesson's central concepts and terminology. Pay special attention to the "Vocabulary Check" exercise and the additional terms and concepts that follow—page references indicate where in the text assignment each term is defined. [Remember: there is a complete Glossary at the end of the text.]

- Take the "Self-Test" to measure the degree to which you are achieving this lesson's learning objectives. Check your answers against the "Answer Key" and review when necessary.

- Follow the suggestions in the "Study Activities" section at the end of this lesson and complete any other activities and projects assigned by your instructor.

Learning Objectives

When you have completed all assignments in this lesson, you should be able to:

1. Define social psychology and list examples of the types of questions explored in this field.

2. Define norms and social roles, and explain the relationship between them.

3. Describe the results of Zimbardo's "prison study" and Milgram's "obedience study," and explain how each illustrates the power of social roles to influence behavior.

4. Describe attribution theory and distinguish between situational and dispositional attributions. Describe and provide examples of the fundamental attribution error, self-serving bias, and the just-world hypothesis.

5. Discuss the benefits as well as several problems associated with using stereotypes. Explain how differences between cultural values and rules may lead to inaccurate negative stereotypes.

6. Define attitudes and explain their relation to behavior.

7. Describe several ways prejudices develop and the effects of prejudicial attitudes on behavior, and explain why prejudicial attitudes are resistant to change.

Overview

This lesson—the first of two on social psychology—identifies some of the principles of social life. It shows how the roles and rules (norms) of social life influence human behavior. Among the more dramatic demonstrations of the importance of social psychology are some famous, yet controversial, research studies (Zimbardo's "prison study" and Milgram's "obedience study"), which are carefully described and evaluated in this lesson. The textbook provides updates and new cross-cultural findings on the Milgram experiments and new assessments of Milgram's paradigm. It also offers Zimbardo's reflections 25 years after his famous study.

The lesson discusses **attribution theory** and defines **fundamental attribution error**, **self-serving bias**, and the **just-world hypothesis**. It shows what **stereotypes** are and can do, and it explains **attitudes**.

There is a thorough section on **prejudice**, including an explanation of why it can be so resistant to change.

The textbook's coverage of social and cultural psychology, in Chapter 8, has been augmented with updated information and the results of cross-cultural research.

Viewing Notes

"Social Psychology" is the first of two video programs on social psychology. It shows how people's behavior is influenced by the social roles they play, by the social norms or rules governing different roles. Experts discuss some of the exciting and controversial research that has been performed by social psychologists.

As you watch the video program, consider the following questions:

1. What are the principal problems, questions, and issues that interest social psychologists?

2. What positive functions do stereotypes serve, and what are some of their negative (dysfunctional) aspects?

3. What are the sources and components of biases and prejudices?

4. What does Jim Sidanius say about the scapegoating theory of how prejudice develops?

5. What role does the concept of "in" groups and "out" groups (of "us" versus "them") play in the development and maintenance of prejudice?

6. Why was it so easy for Marilynn Brewer and her colleagues to create groups in the laboratory who were biased against each other?

7. What means did Brewer's group find that tended to reduce bias and prejudice?

8. Why is attribution theory central to understanding the relationship between beliefs and behavior?

9. How does Lee Ross describe the fundamental attribution error and its significance?

10. How does Bernard Weiner define the self-serving bias?

11. What does the depiction of the Zimbardo "prison study" demonstrate about the power of social roles to influence behavior?

Review Exercises

Vocabulary Check

Match the following key terms and concepts with the appropriate definitions from the list below.

1. ____ attitude (p. 274)

2. ____ attribution theory (p. 272; video)

3. ____ cognitive dissonance (p. 275)

4. ____ fundamental attribution error (p. 272; video)

5. ____ just-world hypothesis (p. 274; video)

6. ____ norms (social) (p. 264)

7. ____ prejudice (p. 290; video)

8. ____ role (p. 264; video)

9. ____ scapegoat (p. 291; video)

10. ____ self-serving bias (p. 273; video)

11. ____ stereotype (p. 289; video)

12. ____ validity effect (p. 276)

a. the tendency of people to take credit for good actions and to excuse or rationalize their mistakes

b. a state of tension that occurs when a person simultaneously holds two cognitions that are psychologically inconsistent, or when a person's belief is inconsistent with his or her behavior

c. the notion that people need to believe that the world is fair and that justice is served, that bad people are punished and good people are rewarded

d. social conventions that regulate human life, including explicit laws and implicit cultural standards

e. a cognitive schema or a summary impression of a group, in which a person believes that all members of the group share a common trait or traits (positive, negative, or neutral)

f. the tendency to overestimate personality factors (dispositions) and underestimate environmental ones (situations) when explaining behavior

g. a powerless target of an individual's or group's prejudice that is made to bear the blame for personal or social problems

h. an unjustified negative attitude toward a group of people or a custom

i. a fairly stable opinion regarding a person, object, or activity, containing a cognitive element (perceptions and beliefs) and an emotional element (positive or negative feelings)

j. the tendency of people to believe that a statement is true or valid simply because it has been repeated many times

k. a given social position that is governed by a set of norms for proper behavior

l. the theory that people are motivated to explain their own and others' behavior by ascribing causes of that behavior to a situation or disposition

Other Key Terms and Concepts

discrimination (pp. 291–298)

entrapment (p. 271)

ethnocentrism (p. 288)

social cognition (p. 272)

social comparison (video)

social identity (p. 288)

social psychology (p. 263)

Completion

Fill each blank with the most appropriate term from the list of answers below.

13. The field of _____ studies people in social contexts, including the influences of _____, _____, and _____ on behavior and cognition.

14. A role is a social _____ that is governed by a set of _____, also called norms.

15. In Zimbardo's _____, students played the roles of _____ and _____.

16. You make a _____ attribution when you regard an action as being caused by something in the environment and a _____ attribution when you regard an action as being caused by something in a person, such as a motive or trait.

17. Stereotypes _____ differences within other groups and _____ differences between groups.

18. The human wish for _____ tends to bring attitudes and behavior into harmony.

19. One of the reasons prejudices are resistant to change is that they provide a _____ in self-esteem and reduced anxiety because they allow people to feel proud of themselves and their own group and superior to others.

accentuate	norms	roles
consistency	position	rules
dispositional	"prison study"	situational
groups	prisoners	social psychology
guards	psychological benefit	underestimate

True-False

Read the following statements carefully and mark each true (T) or false (F).

20. ___ One of the most significant areas studied by social psychologists is the power of social roles to influence how people act and think.

21. ___ Everyone in a society must obey the social rules known as norms, which are the same for everyone, no matter what roles they play.

22. ___ In Milgram's "obedience study," the social role of the people conducting the experiment gave them sufficient authority to override the test subject's instinct to refrain from inflicting pain on a defenseless person.

23. ___ The just-world hypothesis can lead to the dispositional attribution called "blaming the victim," because in a just world good people are rewarded and villains are punished, so someone who is punished may well be a villain and thus deserve punishment.

24. ___ Stereotypes are always wrong.

25. ___ Attitudes are opinions that are easily and regularly changed.

26. ___ People who are the objects of prejudice have usually done something as individuals to create the negative attitudes directed against them.

Short-Answer Questions

As a final review exercise, write brief answers to demonstrate that you are achieving the learning objectives of this lesson.

1. Define social psychology and list examples of the types of questions explored in this field.

2. Define norms and social roles, and explain the relationship between them.

3. Describe the results of Zimbardo's "prison study" and Milgram's "obedience study," and explain how each illustrates the power of social roles to influence behavior.

4. Describe attribution theory and distinguish between situational and dispositional attributions. Describe and provide examples of the fundamental attribution error, self-serving bias, and the just-world hypothesis.

5. Discuss the benefits as well as several problems associated with using stereotypes. Explain how differences between cultural values and rules may lead to inaccurate negative stereotypes.

6. Define attitudes and explain their relation to behavior.

7. Describe several ways prejudices develop and the effects of prejudicial attitudes on behavior, and explain why prejudicial attitudes are resistant to change.

Self-Test

1. Social psychology is **LEAST** likely to explore the relationships between a person's perceptions, attitudes, emotions, and behavior and his or her

    a. dreams.

    b. group.

    c. culture.

    d. relationships.

2. Which of the following are **NOT** major research areas in social psychology?

    a. attitudes and explanations

    b. obedience and conformity

    c. learning and development

    d. cooperation and competition

3. Gender _____ define(s) the "proper" _____ for men and women.

    a. preferences; attire

    b. norms; roles

    c. experiences; attitudes

    d. roles; behavior

4. How many social roles would any one person be expected to play at any one time in contemporary society?

    a. no more than one

    b. two or three

    c. many

    d. as many as there are members of his or her peer group

5. In the Zimbardo "prison study,"
   a. students played prisoners and teachers played guards.
   b. teachers played prisoners and students played guards.
   c. students played both prisoners and guards, but refused to stick to their roles.
   d. students played both prisoners and guards, quickly learned their roles, and played them to the hilt.

6. The experiment in which people were asked to shock people who failed to show progress in learning was the
   a. Zimbardo "prison study."
   b. Milgram "obedience study."
   c. Rosenhan "hospital study."
   d. Asch "conformity study."

7. Taken together, the most important point that Zimbardo's "prison study" and Milgram's "obedience study" make is that
   a. social roles have considerable power to control behavior.
   b. you can "fool some of the people some of the time."
   c. people use physical punishment to achieve their goals.
   d. there is little difference between mental hospitals and prisons.

8. If you tend to believe that salespeople, flight attendants, and others whose jobs require them to be charming and friendly to the public act the way they do because of their personalities, that is an example of
   a. fundamental attribution error.
   b. self-serving bias.
   c. prejudice.
   d. stereotyping.

9. The tendency to take credit for good actions and to excuse or rationalize your mistakes is called

  a. fundamental attribution error.

  b. self-serving bias.

  c. prejudice.

  d. stereotyping.

10. You may know people with the personal belief that all of humanity is subject to forces that reward good people and take away from people who are evil or do not deserve better. This belief is called the

  a. law of diminishing returns.

  b. law of supply and demand.

  c. capitalist theory.

  d. just-world hypothesis.

11. All members of a stereotyped group are thought to

  a. hate the members of other groups.

  b. be much like the members of other groups.

  c. share a common trait or traits.

  d. love and respect all the members of their own group.

12. When people like a particular group, their stereotype of the group's behavior tends to be

  a. accurate.

  b. neutral.

  c. positive.

  d. exaggerated.

13. You believe that Japanese are serious and hardworking and that Hawaiians are fun loving and undependable. This is an example of how stereotypes can

  a. help you deal with actual Japanese or Hawaiian individuals.

  b. create selective perceptions.

  c. lead to dissonance.

  d. emphasize the differences between groups.

14. A stereotype can be particularly divisive when
    a. the members of different groups are from different cultures or religions or countries.
    b. the members of both groups are very much alike.
    c. some individuals are members of both groups.
    d. no one really believes in it.

15. According to psychologists,
    a. attitudes always come before behavior.
    b. behavior always comes before attitudes.
    c. causality works in both directions: attitudes can change behavior and behavior can create new attitudes.
    d. something else has to change both attitudes and behavior.

16. Attitudes and behavior can be brought into harmony by the wish for
    a. cognitive dissonance.
    b. consistency.
    c. convictions.
    d. social cognition.

17. A powerless target of an individual's or a group's prejudice that is made to bear the blame for personal or social problems is called a
    a. victim.
    b. scapegoat.
    c. role model.
    d. stereotype.

18. Which of the following is **NOT** one of the factors making attitudes in general and prejudice in particular so resistant to change.
    a. socialization benefits
    b. the social benefits
    c. the economic benefits
    d. the psychodynamic benefits

19. The first time Larry walks through a Puerto Rican neighborhood, some Puerto Rican teenagers yell and gesture at him aggressively. What is likely to happen to Larry as a result of this incident.

    a. He will experience cognitive dissonance.

    b. He will try to learn more about Puerto Rican territoriality and other values.

    c. He will assume that he was doing something that justifiably upset the teenagers.

    d. He will develop a prejudice toward Puerto Ricans.

Study Activities

These activities challenge you to use your critical thinking and demonstrate how what you are learning can be applied to you and your own life. Choose those activities that interest you most and/or those your instructor assigns.

1. What social roles do you now play, have you played in the past, and do you realistically expect to play in the future? Anyone reading these words is probably filling the role of student. If you're a man, you have a male gender role; if you're a woman, your role is female. You are, or have been, someone's child, and so you have played and may still be playing that role. That is not to say you act like a child, but rather that you behave toward your parents in ways appropriate to that relationship. In that connection, you may also be a parent and have to fill that role in relation to your own children.

    Think of all your roles: at work, in the community, among your friends, in your family. You'll be surprised at how many there are. As you identify them, consider the norms that govern your behavior in each role. How are you supposed to act in each role?

2. Everyone has stereotyped attitudes, positive or negative, toward others. You may regret some of yours, or know they are inaccurate, but find it hard to ignore them. The reading assignment explains this process. For this exercise, take a different approach. Think of stereotypes other people may apply to you. You are a member of a racial or ethnic group. Your appearance, manner of dress, and occupation; the car you drive; the breed of your dog; your neighborhood and place of birth—almost anything can make you subject to being stereotyped. Think of all the things that might make someone think of you as being in a group with "others like you."

    Think of how it feels to be categorized with no regard to who you are as an individual.

Lesson 25

Individuals and Groups

Assignments

For the most systematic coverage of this lesson, we suggest that you complete the assignments in the sequence listed below.

Before viewing the video program:

- Read the "Learning Objectives" and "Overview" for this lesson. Use the Learning Objectives to guide your reading, viewing, and thinking.

- Read the "Viewing Notes" for this lesson.

- Read Chapter 8, "Behavior in Social and Cultural Context," pages 279–288 and 296–301, and review pages 266–268, in the Wade and Tavris text. First, familiarize yourself with its contents by reading the Chapter Outline. As you read, note terms and concepts set in bold or italic type, especially those defined in the margins. Take the Quick Quizzes to check your understanding of material being described and explained.

View the video program, "Conformity, Obedience, and Dissent"

After viewing the video program:

- Briefly note your answers to the questions at the end of the "Viewing Notes."

- Review all reading assignments for this lesson, including the Summary at the end of Chapter 8 in the textbook.

- Complete the "Review Exercises" to strengthen your understanding of this lesson's central concepts and terminology. Pay special attention to the "Vocabulary Check" exercise and the additional terms and concepts that follow—page references indicate where in the text assignment each term is defined. [Remember: there is a complete Glossary at the end of the text.]

- Take the "Self-Test" to measure the degree to which you are achieving this lesson's learning objectives. Check your answers against the "Answer Key" and review when necessary.

- Follow the suggestions in the "Study Activities" section at the end of this lesson and complete any other activities and projects assigned by your instructor.

Learning Objectives

When you have completed all assignments in this lesson, you should be able to:

1. Discuss positive and negative aspects of obedience and conformity.

2. Cite several reasons why people may deny their private beliefs and conform to a group; describe the contributions of Solomon Asch's famous series of studies to the understanding of conformity.

3. Identify factors that discourage people from disobeying and describe key stages in the process of dissent.

4. Explain the extreme form of conformity called groupthink.

5. Describe three common features of groupthink. Examine several specific strategies that may counteract groupthink and encourage better and more creative decision making.

6. Explain and provide examples of diffusion of responsibility, deindividuation, and bystander altruism. Describe social conditions that make these situations more likely to occur.

7. Discuss possible negative consequences of competition, and describe conditions that promote cooperation.

8. Describe the contact hypothesis and list four factors that appear necessary to reduce prejudice between groups.

9. Discuss the debate over human nature and consider the degree to which individuals' behavior is governed by instincts or by basic psychological processes.

Overview

This lesson completes the telecourse's coverage of social psychology by examining **conformity**, **obedience**, and **dissent**. Because all human beings function both as individuals and as members of groups, this topic is particularly significant. The lesson focuses on why people obey orders and conform to group standards and beliefs. It indicates what factors discourage people from disobeying or from dissenting. Both the textbook and the video program examine such influential research in this area as Asch's studies of conformity and Milgram's experiment on obedience to authority.

The features of the process known as **groupthink** are identified. The matter of **diffusion of responsibility** is dealt with, including the social conditions that encourage **deindividuation** and affect **bystander altruism**. The mechanisms of **competition** and **cooperation** are also discussed.

Strategies to break down group prejudice are discussed, concentrating on the **contact hypothesis**.

The lesson examines the debate over the relative importance of human nature and basic psychological processes in determining human behavior.

Viewing Notes

This video program, entitled "Conformity, Obedience, and Dissent," examines why and how people conform to group pressure, obey authority, or follow their own conscience. Both the negative and positive aspects of these psychological processes are described and analyzed.

As you watch the video program, consider the following questions:

1. Under what circumstances is conformity most likely to occur?

2. What is the psychological basis for conformity?

3. How did Solomon Asch's classic experiments reveal the power of group dynamics to compel conformity, even if it means the conforming individual must deny the evidence of his or her own senses?

4. What are some of the advantages of conformity, both to the individual and to society?

5. What does Stanley Milgram's experiment tell us about ordinary people's willingness to obey authority, even if it means harming another person?

6. What does research by psychologists Barry Collins and David Levy reveal about how people view dissent?

7. What are the research findings about the role of leadership in group processes?

Review Exercises

Vocabulary Check

Match the following key terms and concepts with the appropriate definitions from the list below.

1. ___ altruism (p. 285)
2. ___ conformity (p. 279; video)
3. ___ contact hypothesis (p. 297)
4. ___ deindividuation (p. 283)
5. ___ diffusion of responsibility (pp. 282–283)
6. ___ entrapment (p. 271)
7. ___ groupthink (p. 281)
8. ___ obedience (pp. 266–272; video)
9. ___ routinization (p. 270)
10. ___ social loafing (p. 282)

a. in close-knit groups, the tendency for all members to think alike and to suppress dissent and disagreement

b. the willingness to take selfless or dangerous action on behalf of others

c. the idea that the best way to reduce group prejudice and stereotyping is simply for members of opposing groups to get to know one another better

d. behavior or attitudes that occur as a result of real or imagined group pressure

e. the process of defining an activity in terms of routine duties and roles so that one's behavior becomes normalized, a job to be done, and there is little opportunity to raise doubts or ethical questions

f. the tendency of group members, under some conditions, to reduce their efforts; one result of diffusion of responsibility

g. a gradual process in which individuals escalate their commitment to a course of action to justify their investment of time, money, or effort

h. behavior performed while following an order from someone in authority

i. in groups or crowds, the loss of awareness of one's own individuality; in varying degrees, a person feels indistinguishable from others

j. in organized or anonymous groups, the tendency of members to avoid taking responsibility for actions or decisions, assuming others will do it

Other Key Terms and Concepts

Asch's classic experiments
(pp. 279–280; video)

bystander apathy (p. 282)

competition (p. 289)

cooperation (pp. 297–298)

crimes of obedience (p. 270)

dissent (p. 285; video)

Completion

Fill each blank with the most appropriate term from the list of answers below.

11. In explaining their actions, people often _____ conformity but _____ obedience.

12. Among the reasons people will deny their private beliefs and conform to a group are _____, _____, _____, _____, and _____.

13. Factors that discourage people from disobeying include _____, _____, and _____.

14. Polarization doesn't mean that the group becomes split between two poles of opinion, but that the group's _____ decision is more extreme than most of its members' individual opinions would be.

15. It has been explained that _____ occurs when a group's need for agreement overwhelms its need to make the wisest decision, and when the members' needs to be liked and accepted overwhelm their ability to disagree with a bad decision.

16. When individual members of a group are not responsible or accountable for the work they do, or when they feel working harder would only duplicate their colleagues' efforts, _____ may result.

17. Competition and cooperation have powerful effects on _____, _____, and _____.

18. One of the factors necessary to reduce prejudice between groups is giving the members of both groups opportunities to _____.

19. In the view of social psychologists, it is not so much that human nature or instincts determine behavior, but that basic psychological processes [such as _____, _____, _____, and _____] provide the capacity for a variety of behaviors—war or peace, aggression or altruism.

attitudes	the desire to be accurate	lacking a language of protest
average	embarrassment	personality
competition	embrace	roles
conformity	entrapment	social loafing
deindividuation	group relations	socialize informally
deny	groupthink	the wish to be liked
the desire for personal gain	identification with the group	

True-False

Read the following statements carefully and mark each true (T) or false (F).

20. ____ Obedience and conformity are basic social processes that are necessary in all human societies.

21. ____ Research shows that real or imagined group pressure can be strong enough to make people deny their private beliefs, agree with silly notions, and do things they would never do on their own.

22. ____ Many people do not disobey, even when they know the orders are foolish or wrong, because they don't know how to stand up to authority; they literally lack the words to protest without embarrassment.

23. ____ In jury deliberations, the verdict initially favored by the majority is usually the one that eventually wins, as group polarization would suggest.

24. ____ One of the forces sustaining groupthink is the desire of members to preserve harmony and stay in the good graces of the leader.

25. ____ Every stage in a bystander's decision to help in a crisis also applies to an individual's decision to protest wrongdoing.

26. ____ Tests of the contact hypothesis have never shown that getting to know one another made members of opposing groups get along any better.

27. ____ Basic psychological processes are neutral and cannot provide the capacity for negative behavior such as aggression, cruelty, and war.

Short-Answer Questions

As a final review exercise, write brief answers to demonstrate that you are achieving the learning objectives of this lesson.

1.   Discuss positive and negative aspects of obedience and conformity.

2.   Cite several reasons why people may deny their private beliefs and conform to a group; describe the contributions of Solomon Asch's famous series of studies to the understanding of conformity.

3.   Identify factors that discourage people from disobeying and describe key stages in the process of dissent.

4.   Explain the extreme form of conformity called groupthink.

5.   Describe three common features of groupthink. Examine several specific strategies that may counteract groupthink and encourage better and more creative decision making.

6.   Explain and provide examples of diffusion of responsibility, deindividuation, and bystander altruism. Describe social conditions that make these situations more likely to occur.

7.   Discuss possible negative consequences of competition, and describe conditions that promote cooperation.

8.   Describe the contact hypothesis and list four factors that appear necessary to reduce prejudice between groups.

9.   Discuss the debate over human nature and consider the degree to which individuals' behavior is governed by instincts or by basic psychological processes.

Self Test

1. Obedience is

    a. always useful to the obedient person and to society.

    b. always harmful to the obedient person and to society.

    c. not always harmful or bad, but can be necessary for the group.

    d. a behavior into which the average person must be tricked or coerced.

2. When people conform to unspoken rules, they tend to believe they are doing so

    a. under duress and coercion.

    b. of their own free will.

    c. out of patriotism.

    d. as an act of protest.

3. Which of the following is **NOT** one of the reasons people are willing to deny their private beliefs and conform to a group.

    a. identification with the group

    b. desire for personal gain

    c. mindlessness

    d. high self-esteem

4. People who conform tend to have personalities marked by

    a. self-assurance.

    b. a strong need for social approval.

    c. flexibility.

    d. a desire to stand out.

5. Someone who was a subject in one of Solomon Asch's original studies of conformity explains he did conform and how he felt. Because he behaved the way most of the subjects did, he reports that he

    a. did not conform at all and was proud of not having done so.

    b. did not conform at all, though he felt a little funny about it.

    c. conformed on some trials, though he felt uncertain when he did so.

    d. conformed on all of the trials and felt resentful that he was forced to do so.

6. Some people are discouraged from disobeying orders because they feel that to disobey would be

    a. rude.

    b. extremist.

    c. self-centered.

    d. ungrateful.

7. The process whereby individuals escalate their commitment to a course of action to justify what they've already invested in it is called

    a. deindividuation.

    b. reactance.

    c. entrapment.

    d. mindlessness.

8. In _____, the group's need for total agreement overwhelms its need to make the wisest decision.

    a. groupthink

    b. diffusion of responsibility

    c. conformity

    d. group polarization

9. Which of the following is **NOT** one of the identifiable features of groupthink?

    a.   preserving harmony and staying in the leader's good graces

    b.   encouraging innovative ideas that will strengthen the group

    c.   avoiding disagreements that will make one's friends look bad

    d.   suppressing dissent and avoiding getting outside information that might challenge the group's views

10. _____ are disruptive to a group, but they force the group to become aware of other ideas and other solutions.

    a.   Leaders

    b.   Conformists

    c.   Dissenters

    d.   Scapegoats

11. The most extreme condition of diffused responsibility is

    a.   deindividuation.

    b.   groupthink.

    c.   ethnocentrism.

    d.   bystander altruism.

12. Social psychologists emphasize that _____ is not simply a spontaneous or selfless expression of a desire to help; there are social conditions that make it more likely to occur.

    a.   reactance

    b.   altruism

    c.   deindividuation

    d.   conformity

13. A major psychological hazard of competition is that

    a.   you may lose.

    b.   you may win once, but never again.

    c.   when winning is everything, it is no longer any fun to come in second or even to play the game.

    d.   if you win too often, no one will want to play with you again.

14. "Us-them" thinking is one consequence of
    a. obedience.

    b. groupthink.

    c. cooperation.

    d. competition.

15. Which of the following is **NOT** one of the four conditions necessary to reduce prejudice and conflict?
    a. Both sides must cooperate.

    b. Both sides must be of the same race or ethnic group.

    c. Both sides must have equal status and equal economic standing.

    d. Both sides must believe they have the moral, legal, and economic support of authorities.

16. The _____ method has been used to get groups that are prejudiced against one another to interact and learn to trust one another; it involves working on a shared task that requires cooperation among many individuals from both groups.
    a. jigsaw

    b. leniency

    c. groupthink

    d. obedience

17. Which of the following is **NOT** one of the basic psychological processes that provide the capacity for aggression or altruism, war or peace?
    a. conformity to one's group and obedience to authority

    b. self-realization

    c. deindividuation

    d. entrapment

Study Activities

The following activity challenges you to use your critical thinking and demonstrate how what you are learning can be applied to you and your own life. Try this activity and/or those your instructor assigns.

Have you ever been involved in group decision making? Have you detected any of the characteristics of groupthink? Have you ever found yourself in a crowd, or worse, a mob, in which everyone seemed to be deindividuated, losing their sense of themselves as individuals as they got caught up in the excitement, enthusiasm, or anger of the group? Have you ever had to choose between obedience to authority or conformity to the group and assertion of your own ideas and individuality? How did you act?

You probably are able to answer all of the preceding questions with ease. All of us have had these experiences. You needn't have been the member of a lynch mob to have experienced deindividuation. Students at a pep rally or any fans at a big game can mindlessly lose themselves in support of one side.

Survey your experience for instances of your personal involvement in situations and social psychological processes discussed in this lesson. Try to think about your behavior objectively, seeing yourself as the subject of this highly informal investigation. Try to identify positive and negative aspects of what you experienced. Concentrate on how you felt—satisfied, proud, embarrassed, suppressed, frustrated, angry, excited, withdrawn, and so on—in group situations in which pressure was placed upon you to conform. Moreover, in recalling such situations, try to remember if you were unaware that forces were compelling you to conform and/or obey. If you have trouble identifying negative feelings, it could mean you had positive or neutral feelings and were consciously or unconsciously conforming and/or obeying.

As you engage in this exercise, think to what degree your individual nature or social circumstances and psychological processes shaped your attitudes and behavior.

Lesson 26

Issues in Psychology

Assignments

For the most systematic coverage of this lesson, we suggest that you complete the assignments in the sequence listed below.

Before viewing the video program:

- Read the "Learning Objectives" and "Overview" for this lesson. Use the Learning Objectives to guide your reading, viewing, and thinking.

- Read the "Viewing Notes" for this lesson.

- Read Epilogue, "Taking Psychology with You," in the Wade and Tavris textbook. First, familiarize yourself with its contents by reading the Chapter Outline. As you read, note terms and concepts set in bold or italic type, especially those defined in the margins. Take the Quick Quizzes to check your understanding of material being described and explained.

View the video program, "Issues in Psychology"

After viewing the video program:

- Briefly note your answers to the questions at the end of the "Viewing Notes."

- Review all reading assignments for this lesson.

- Complete the "Review Exercises" to strengthen your understanding of this lesson's central concepts and terminology.

- Take the "Self-Test" to measure the degree to which you are achieving this lesson's learning objectives. Check your answers against the "Answer Key" and review when necessary.

- Follow the suggestions in the "Study Activities" section at the end of this lesson and complete any other activities and projects assigned by your instructor.

Learning Objectives

When you have completed all assignments in this lesson, you should be able to:

1. Describe the "five strands of human experience" and explain the role they can play in one's life.

2. Explain the importance of psychology to one's life.

3. Be receptive to the possibility that the findings of psychology may be of use in dealing with personal and social problems, but be skeptical about popular and unsubstantiated psychological conclusions.

4. Discuss how the field of psychology is in a constant state of change as new research findings are reported.

Overview

An overview of this lesson is really an overview of the entire telecourse *Psychology: The Study of Human Behavior*.

Both the video program and the text reading assignment are devoted to conclusions and insights based upon the material covered in the other 25 lessons.

This lesson discusses the issues in psychology, the unsettled questions that research and new theories are confronting. It also discusses what you, as a consumer of psychological knowledge who is just completing this survey of psychology, can be expected to take away with you to apply to your real-world problems.

The so-called **five strands of human experience**, the basic factors underlying all psychological theories and methods, are defined and described. The video lesson and text remind us that psychology is never a completed exercise; psychologists never stop trying to discover, to clarify, and to improve their understanding of what it means to be human.

Viewing Notes

"Issues in Psychology" is the final video program in this telecourse. It provides viewers an opportunity to consider how all the things learned earlier fit together and can be applied to current issues in the field.

The program includes an in-studio discussion in which leading psychologists, representing a variety of theoretical and research perspectives, examine major issues facing the field of psychology.

Review Exercises

Completion

Fill each blank with the most appropriate term from the list of answers below.

1. The five strands of human experience are _____, _____, _____, _____, and _____.

2. Psychology can be of long-lasting personal value in dealing with such common real-world problems as _____ and _____.

3. Don't confuse psychological findings based on _____ methods with unsubstantiated _____.

4. Because science is an ongoing process of _____ and _____, existing knowledge is always subject to refinement and change.

biological influences	learning influences	research
cognitive influences	pop psychology	scientific
coping with interpersonal relations	psychodynamic influences	social and cultural influences
dealing with job stress	reevaluation of existing theories	

True-False

Read the following statements carefully and mark each true (T) or false (F).

5. ___ Each of the five strands of human existence is a separate force that operates independently of the other four.

6. ___ Psychology is of real importance in your life only if you have serious psychological problems or a particularly chaotic social life.

7. ___ Much of so-called pop psychology is as valid, reliable, and useful as anything academic psychologists write about in professional journals.

8. ___ Psychology has made most of its important discoveries, and most research psychologists now concentrate on consolidating and fine tuning the multitude of established, agreed-upon theories.

Short-Answer Questions

As a final review exercise, write brief answers to demonstrate that you are achieving the learning objectives of this lesson.

1. Describe the "five strands of human experience" and explain the role they can play in one's life.

2. Explain the importance of psychology to one's life.

3. Be receptive to the possibility that the findings of psychology may be of use in dealing with personal and social problems, but be skeptical about popular and unsubstantiated psychological conclusions.

4. Discuss how the field of psychology is in a constant state of change as new research findings are reported.

Self-Test

1. Which of the five strands of human experience is concerned with your ability to make attributions?

    a.   biological influences

    b.   cognitive influences

    c.   learning influences

    d.   social and cultural influences

2. Which of the five strands of human experience deals with the contingencies and consequences governing your behavior and that of others?

    a.   cognitive influences

    b.   psychodynamic influences

    c.   social and cultural influences

    d.   learning influences

3. To discover how significant and valuable psychology can be in your life; you must

    a.   find someone to select those aspects of psychological knowledge that can be of benefit to you.

    b.   select those aspects of psychological knowledge that can be of benefit to you.

    c.   undergo psychotherapy.

    d.   become a psychologist.

4. For any given disorder or problem in living, psychology

    a.   usually offers a specific theory and technique.

    b.   probably has no answer whatever.

    c.   usually offers several different approaches.

    d.   has a theory, but no technique for dealing with it.

5. The hallmark of the psychological approach to understanding and dealing with problems—an approach that distinguishes it from most popular and unsubstantiated pseudopsychology—might be simply stated as

    a. critical thinking.

    b. deep conviction.

    c. trusting followers.

    d. lack of controversy.

Study Activities

This activity challenges you to use your critical thinking and demonstrate how what you are learning can be applied to you and your own life. Try this activity or those that your instructor assigns.

In a sense this entire lesson is a study activity for the entire telecourse. The purpose of the lesson is to review what you have studied. It invites you to consider how to take what you've learned away with you, how to apply it to your real-world problems and needs. It challenges you to employ the critical thinking skills you've been developing throughout the course in your everyday life.

Rather than a separate study activity, you would be best served to read the text assignment, the book's Epilogue, and follow the suggestions of authors Carole Wade and Carol Tavris. They have prepared you to finish this course and feel confident enough to use what you've learned. Following the suggestions in their Epilogue can be the real test of their success ... and yours.

Answer Key

Lesson 1   What Is Psychology?

Review Exercises

Vocabulary Check

1. l	6. b	11. d
2. h	7. i	12. e
3. a	8. c	13. k
4. j	9. m	
5. g	10. f	

Completion

14. describe, modify or control, predict, understand (in any order)
15. common sense
16. psychiatry
17. B. F. Skinner, John B. Watson (in any order)
18. Sigmund Freud
19. basic psychology, applied psychology
20. social, industrial/organizational
21. feminist
22. constructive, creative (in any order)

True-False

23. F	27. T	31. F
24. F	28. F	32. F
25. T	29. T	33. T
26. F	30. T	

Self-Test

[Page numbers refer to the Wade and Tavris text.]

1. c (Objective 1; page 2; video program)
2. c (Objective 1; page 14)
3. b (Objective 1; page 13)
4. d (Objective 1; pages 15–16)
5. d (Objective 2; pages 3–4)
6. b (Objective 3; page 18)
7. c (Objective 3; page 19)
8. b (Objective 3; page 14)
9. a (Objective 3; pages 20–21)
10. c (Objective 3; page 27; video program)
11. d (Objective 4; page 23)
12. b (Objective 4; page 23)
13. c (Objective 4; page 25)
14. c (Objective 4; page 23)
15. a (Objective 5; page 5)
16. b (Objective 5; page 7)
17. c (Objective 5; page 8)

Lesson 2   How Psychologists Know What They Know

Review Exercises

Vocabulary Check

1. g
2. m
3. o
4. d
5. i

6. f
7. a
8. k
9. n
10. b

11. e
12. l
13. j
14. h
15. c

Completion

16. confirmation bias
17. openness, precision, reliance on empirical evidence, skepticism, willingness to make "risky predictions" (in any order)
18. naturalistic observation, laboratory observation
19. population
20. psychological
21. causation
22. control, causes
23. independent variable, dependent variable
24. experimenter effects
25. laboratory
26. meta-analysis
27. ethical

True-False

28. F
29. T
30. F
31. T

32. F
33. T
34. T
35. F

36. F
37. T
38. F

Self-Test

[Page numbers refer to the Wade and Tavris text.]

1. c (Objective 1; page 34)
2. b (Objective 1; page 39; video program)
3. b (Objective 1; page 35)
4. c (Objective 1; pages 35–36)
5. c (Objective 2; page 38)
6. b (Objective 2; page 39)
7. a (Objective 2; page 43)
8. a (Objective 2; page 41)
9. a (Objective 3; page 45)
10. d (Objective 3; page 46)
11. c (Objective 3; page 46)
12. b (Objective 4; page 48)
13. c (Objective 4; page 48)
14. b (Objective 5; pages 48–49)
15. a (Objective 5; page 48)
16. c (Objective 5; page 50)
17. c (Objective 5; page 51)
18. d (Objective 5; page 51; video program)
19. b (Objective 6; pages 55–57)
20. d (Objective 6; page 55)
21. c (Objective 6; page 57)
22. b (Objective 7; page 59)
23. d (Objective 7; page 59)
24. c (Objective 7; page 60)

Lesson 3   The Biology of Behavior

Review Exercises

Vocabulary Check

1. n
2. e
3. i
4. h
5. l

6. m
7. d
8. g
9. k
10. a

11. c
12. b
13. f
14. j

Completion

15. central
16. autonomic
17. somatic
18. biofeedback
19. sympathetic, parasympathetic
20. glial, neurons
21. dendrites, cell
22. myelin sheath
23. neurotransmitters
24. synaptic vesicles
25. endorphins, heroin
26. endocrine glands, bloodstream
27. melatonin
28. androgens, estrogens

True-False

29. F
30. T
31. F
32. T

33. F
34. F
35. T
36. F

37. T
38. F
39. T

Self-Test

[Page numbers refer to the Wade and Tavris text.]

1. b (Objective 1; page 100; video program)
2. a (Objective 1; page 100)
3. d (Objective 1; page 101)
4. c (Objective 1; page 101)
5. d (Objective 2; page 102)
6. c (Objective 2; page 102)
7. a (Objective 2; page 102)
8. b (Objective 2; page 102)
9. c (Objective 3; page 106)
10. c (Objective 3; page 105; video program)
11. b (Objective 3; page 105; video program)
12. a (Objective 3; page 105; video program)
13. d (Objective 3; page 105; video program)
14. b (Objective 3; page 107; video program)
15. a (Objective 4; page 109; video program)
16. c (Objective 4; page 109; video program)
17. d (Objective 4; page 106)
18. c (Objective 4; page 109)
19. b (Objective 4; page 110)
20. a (Objective 4; page 109)
21. b (Objective 5; page 111; video program)
22. a (Objective 5; page 111; video program)
23. d (Objective 5; video program)
24. c (Objective 5; page 111; video program)
25. b (Objective 5; page 111)

Lesson 4   The Brain-Mind Connection

Review Exercises

Vocabulary Check

1. d
2. i
3. l
4. a
5. m

6. f
7. h
8. n
9. c
10. j

11. g
12. b
13. e
14. o
15. k

Completion

16. electrodes
17. positron-emission tomography (PET scan), magnetic resonance imaging (MRI)
18. medulla, pons (in any order), reticular activating, cerebellum
19. hindbrain, midbrain (in any order), forebrain
20. cerebral cortex
21. frontal
22. left, right, language
23. localization of function, holistic
24. human males and females
25. environmental, social (in any order)

True-False

26. F
27. T
28. F
29. T

30. T
31. F
32. F
33. F

34. T
35. T

Self-Test

[Page numbers refer to the Wade and Tavris text.]

1. a (Objective 1; page 113)
2. c (Objective 1; page 114; video program)
3. d (Objective 1; page 114; video program)
4. c (Objective 2; page 117)
5. d (Objective 2; page 117)
6. a (Objective 3; pages 117–118)
7. c (Objective 3; page 118; video program)
8. b (Objective 3; page 119)
9. b (Objective 3; page 119)
10. d (Objective 4; page 120)
11. b (Objective 4; page 120)
12. c (Objective 4; page 120)
13. a (Objective 4; page 121)
14. d (Objective 5; page 125)
15. c (Objective 5; pages 125–126)
16. b (Objective 5; page 127)
17. b (Objective 6; page 116; video program)
18. c (Objective 6; page 116)
19. a (Objective 6; page 107; video program)
20. b (Objective 7; video program)
21. d (Objective 7; page 130)
22. b (Objective 7; page 132)
23. d (Objective 7; page 133)
24. b (Objective 7; page 132)

Lesson 5   Body Rhythms and Mental States

Review Exercises

Vocabulary Check

1. j	6. n	11. c
2. b	7. d	12. m
3. h	8. o	13. f
4. g	9. e	14. a
5. l	10. i	15. k

Completion

16. desynchronization
17. emotional, mental (in any order)
18. delta, alpha
19. problem solving
20. information-processing
21. activation-synthesis
22. stimulants, depressants
23. physical condition, mental set
24. hypnosis
25. consciousness, dissociation, hidden observer

True-False

26. T	31. F	36. F
27. F	32. T	37. F
28. F	33. F	38. F
29. T	34. T	39. T
30. F	35. F	

Self-Test

[Page numbers refer to the Wade and Tavris text.]

1. a (Objective 1; page 140)
2. d (Objective 1; page 142)
3. c (Objective 1; page 142)
4. d (Objective 2; page 151)
5. c (Objective 2; page 152; video program)
6. b (Objective 2; page 152; video program)
7. b (Objective 3; pages 152, 170; video program)
8. d (Objective 3; page 154)
9. a (Objective 3; page 155)
10. b (Objective 3; page 156; video program)
11. c (Objective 3; page 157; video program)
12. d (Objective 4; page 161)
13. b (Objective 4; pages 161–162)
14. d (Objective 4; pages 161–162)
15. c (Objective 4; pages 161–162)
16. c (Objective 4; pages 162–163)
17. b (Objective 5; pages 165–166)
18. c (Objective 5; page 166)
19. d (Objective 5; page 165)
20. c (Objective 6; page 170)
21. b (Objective 6; page 170)
22. d (Objective 6; page 173)

Lesson 6   Sensation and Perception

Review Exercises

Vocabulary Check

1. j
2. a
3. i
4. k
5. n

6. l
7. b
8. g
9. c
10. f

11. m
12. o
13. e
14. h
15. d

Completion

16. organs, receptors
17. transduction
18. signal detection
19. selective attention
20. retina, rods, cones
21. loudness, pitch, timbre (in any order)
22. perceptual constancy
23. perceptual set
24. culture
25. subliminal perception

True-False

26. F
27. T
28. T
29. T
30. F

31. F
32. F
33. T
34. F
35. F

36. F
37. T
38. F

Self-Test

[Page numbers refer to the Wade and Tavris text.]

1. b (Objective 1; pages 179–180)
2. d (Objective 1; page 180)
3. c (Objective 1; page 180; video program)
4. d (Objective 2; page 180)
5. b (Objective 2; page 181; video program)
6. d (Objective 3; page 186)
7. b (Objective 3; page 187)
8. c (Objective 3; page 187)
9. a (Objective 4; pages 188, 201)
10. c (Objective 4; pages 188, 201)
11. b (Objective 4; page 205)
12. c (Objective 4; page 210)
13. b (Objective 4; page 209)
14. b (Objective 5; pages 198–199; video program)
15. b (Objective 5; pages 197–198)
16. b (Objective 5; pages 215–216)
17. d (Objective 6; pages 213–214; video program)
18. b (Objective 6; page 214; video program)
19. c (Objective 6; pages 212–213)
20. b (Objective 7; page 217)
21. b (Objective 7; page 218)

Lesson 7 Learning

Review Exercises

Vocabulary Check

1. e
2. d
3. b
4. j
5. i

6. h
7. n
8. a
9. c
10. f

11. l
12. g
13. m
14. k

Completion

15. Pavlovian
16. extinction
17. operant
18. reinforcer
19. intermittent
20. punishment
21. behavior modification
22. token economy
23. biological constraints on learning
24. extrinsic
25. observational learning
26. cognitive

True-False

27. F
28. T
29. F
30. F

31. F
32. T
33. F
34. F

35. T
36. T
37. F

Self-Test

[Page numbers refer to the Wade and Tavris text.]

1. b (Objective 1; page 226; video program)
2. c (Objective 1; page 229)
3. d (Objective 1; page 233)
4. a (Objective 2; page 236)
5. b (Objective 2; page 238; video program)
6. c (Objective 2; pages 240–242; video program)
7. c (Objective 3; page 237)
8. a (Objective 3; page 242)
9. b (Objective 3; page 243)
10. b (Objective 4; pages 247–250)
11. c (Objective 4; page 250)
12. d (Objective 5; page 247; video program)
13. b (Objective 5; video program)
14. d (Objective 5; pages 247–252)
15. c (Objective 6; page 251; video program)
16. b (Objective 6; pages 251–252; video program)
17. a (Objective 6; pages 251–252)
18. c (Objective 7; page 256)
19. c (Objective 7; pages 253–254)
20. d (Objective 8; page 257)
21. c (Objective 8; page 257)

Lesson 8   Memory

Review Exercises

Vocabulary Check

1. o	6. h	11. b
2. d	7. l	12. i
3. g	8. n	13. f
4. k	9. e	14. m
5. c	10. j	15. a

Completion

16. encoding, retrieval, storage (in any order)
17. tip-of-the-tongue state (or phenomenon)
18. biochemistry, neurons, structure (in any order)
19. mnemonic
20. neurons
21. retain (or store), retrieve (in any order)
22. schema
23. recency
24. three-box; long-term, sensory, short-term (in any order)
25. flashbulb
26. recovered-memory, false-memory
27. computer

True-False

28. T	32. F	36. F
29. F	33. T	37. T
30. T	34. T	
31. F	35. T	

Self-Test

[Page numbers refer to the Wade and Tavris text.]

1. c (Objective 1; video program)
2. d (Objective 1; pages 348, 357–358)
3. b (Objective 2; pages 366–367)
4. a (Objective 2; page 357)
5. d (Objective 3; page 358)
6. a (Objective 3; page 359)
7. b (Objective 3; page 368)
8. b (Objective 3; pages 367–368)
9. a (Objective 3; page 357)
10. b (Objective 4; page 364)
11. c (Objective 4; pages 352–354; video program)
12. a (Objective 5; page 377)
13. c (Objective 5; page 378)
14. b (Objective 6; page 367)
15. d (Objective 6; page 369)
16. c (Objective 6; page 385)
17. c (Objective 7; page 370; video program)
18. b (Objective 7; pages 370–374; video program)
19. c (Objective 7; pages 373–374; video program)
20. d (Objective 8; pages 380–381)
21. T (Objective 8; video program)
22. F (Objective 8; pages 351–352)
23. F (Objective 8; video program)

Lesson 9   Decision Making and Problem Solving

Review Exercises

Vocabulary Check

1. b
2. i
3. n
4. a
5. m
6. j
7. k
8. f
9. g
10. e
11. c
12. h
13. d
14. l

Completion

15. concept
16. propositions
17. subconscious
18. deductive
19. dialectical
20. irrationality
21. availability heuristic
22. recognizing (or identifying), defining, devising (or selecting), executing (or mastering), evaluating (or monitoring)
23. algorithms, heuristics
24. mental set
25. divergent, convergent
26. confidence, curiosity, independence, nonconformity, persistence (in any order)

True-False

27. F
28. T
29. F
30. F
31. T
32. F
33. F
34. T
35. T
36. F
37. F

Self-Test

[Page numbers refer to the Wade and Tavris text.]

1. b (Objective 1; page 306)
2. c (Objective 1; page 306)
3. a (Objective 2; page 308)
4. c (Objective 2; page 308)
5. d (Objective 3; page 310)
6. c (Objective 3; page 311)
7. a (Objective 3; page 310; video program)
8. c (Objective 4; page 312)
9. b (Objective 4; page 313)
10. c (Objective 5; page 316; video program)
11. c (Objective 5; page 317; video program)
12. b (Objective 6; page 330)
13. a (Objective 6; page 330; video program)
14. b (Objective 6; page 331; video program)
15. b (Objective 7; page 310)
16. a (Objective 7; page 312)
17. c (Objective 7; page 312)
18. b (Objective 8; page 320)
19. d (Objective 9; page 341)
20. c (Objective 9; page 341)
21. b (Objective 9; video program)
22. d (Objective 9; page 341)

Lesson 10   Language

Review Exercises

Vocabulary Check

1. d	6. e	11. k
2. j	7. h	12. a
3. m	8. b	13. c
4. i	9. f	
5. g	10. l	

Completion

14. displacement, meaningfulness, productivity (in any order)
15. surface structure, deep structure
16. grammar
17. nonverbal cues
18. theory of linguistic relativity; perception, thought (in any order)
19. nonhuman animals
20. babbling phase
21. telegraphic speech
22. biological readiness, social experience (interaction) [in any order]
23. parentese (baby talk)
24. close human relationships, practice in conversation (in any order)

True-False

25. F	29. T	33. F
26. T	30. F	34. T
27. F	31. T	35. F
28. F	32. T	

Self-Test

[Page numbers refer to the Wade and Tavris text.]

1. c (Objective 1; page 337; video program)
2. c (Objective 1; page 337; video program)
3. b (Objective 1; pages 73, 504)
4. a (Objective 1; page 73)
5. d (Objective 2; page 338; video program)
6. b (Objective 2; page 338)
7. c (Objective 2; page 339; video program)
8. d (Objective 3; telecourse student guide, page 145; video program)
9. b (Objective 3; video program)
10. d (Objective 3; video program)
11. c (Objective 4; pages 504–505; video program)
12. b (Objective 4; page 74)
13. b (Objective 4; page 76; video program)
14. b (Objective 5; page 73; video program)
15. a (Objective 5; page 74)
16. d (Objective 5; page 76)
17. a (Objective 5; page 76; video program)

Lesson 11   Emotion

Review Exercises

Vocabulary Check

1. f
2. e
3. h
4. l

5. c
6. a
7. g
8. b

9. j
10. k
11. i
12. d

Completion

13. body , culture, mind (in any order)
14. facial feedback
15. epinephrine, norepinephrine (in any order); arousal
16. limbic, hypothalamus
17. two-factor, physiological arousal, cognitive interpretation
18. attributions
19. primary, secondary
20. display rules
21. express
22. aggressive action

True-False

23. T
24. T
25. F
26. T

27. F
28. F
29. T
30. F

31. T
32. F
33. F

Self-Test

[Page numbers refer to the Wade and Tavris text.]

1. b (Objective 1; page 392)
2. c (Objective 1; page 401)
3. b (Objective 1; pages 398–399)
4. d (Objective 2; page 393; video program)
5. b (Objective 2; page 394)
6. c (Objective 2; video program)
7. c (Objective 3; page 398)
8. b (Objective 3; pages 398–399)
9. a (Objective 3; pages 416–417; video program)
10. b (Objective 4; pages 396–398)
11. c (Objective 4; page 398)
12. b (Objective 4; pages 396–397)
13. d (Objective 5; pages 400–405)
14. b (Objective 6; page 406)
15. a (Objective 6; page 406)
16. d (Objective 6; page 411)
17. b (Objective 7; pages 409–410)
18. c (Objective 7; page 410)
19. b (Objective 7; page 410)
20. b (Objective 8; pages 412–414)
21. c (Objective 8; page 415)

Lesson 12   Motivation

Review Exercises

Vocabulary Check

1. n
2. a
3. m
4. l
5. d

6. o
7. j
8. f
9. h
10. b

11. k
12. i
13. e
14. c
15. g

Completion

16. emotion, motivation (in any order)
17. approach-approach, approach-avoidance
18. drive theory
19. set-point
20. curiosity
21. cognitive dissonance
22. contact comfort
23. self-fulfilling prophecy
24. self-efficacy
25. fame, money (in any order); curiosity, happiness, intellectual satisfaction (in any order)
26. simultaneously

True-False

27. F
28. T
29. F
30. T

31. F
32. T
33. T
34. F

35. F
36. T
37. F

Self-Test

[Page numbers refer to the Wade and Tavris text.]

1. a (Objective 1; page 422)
2. b (Objective 1; page 421; video program)
3. b (Objective 2; page 450)
4. c (Objective 2; page 449)
5. d (Objective 2; page 450)
6. c (Objective 3; page 421)
7. c (Objective 3; page 421; video program)
8. d (Objective 4; page 84)
9. a (Objective 4; page 84)
10. c (Objective 5; page 70)
11. d (Objective 5; page 71)
12. b (Objective 6; page 321)
13. c (Objective 6; page 323)
14. a (Objective 7; page 429)
15. c (Objective 8; pages 447–448)
16. a (Objective 9; pages 341, 452)
17. d (Objective 9; page 341; video program)
18. c (Objective 9; page 451; video program)
19. d (Objective 10; video program)

Lesson 13   Gender and Relationships

Review Exercises

Vocabulary Check

1. i	6. h	11. n
2. m	7. a	12. g
3. e	8. c	13. d
4. l	9. f	14. k
5. b	10. j	

Completion

15. testosterone; learning, sociocultural factors (in any order)
16. learn
17. normal
18. varieties
19. behavior, motives
20. companionate, passionate (in any order)
21. emotionally detached, genitally focused (in any order); love and attachment
22. sociobiology
23. gender schema

True-False

24. F	28. F	32. F
25. T	29. T	33. T
26. F	30. T	34. F
27. F	31. F	

Self-Test

1. c (Objective 1; page 432)
2. d (Objective 1; page 432)
3. c (Objective 1; page 432)
4. a (Objective 2; pages 436–437; video program)
5. b (Objective 2; pages 436–437)
6. d (Objective 2; page 440)
7. b (Objective 3; pages 77–78, 434)
8. b (Objective 3; page 79)
9. c (Objective 3; page 437)
10. c (Objective 3; page 436)
11. d (Objective 4; pages 436–437)
12. b (Objective 4; page 438; video program)
13. c (Objective 4; page 438)
14. d (Objective 4; pages 514–515)
15. b (Objective 5; page 426)
16. a (Objective 5; page 426)
17. c (Objective 5; pages 422, 426)
18. a (Objective 5; pages 427–428)
19. b (Objective 5; pages 426–427)

Lesson 14   Theories of the Person and Personality

Review Exercises

Vocabulary Check

1. c
2. j
3. f
4. h

5. e
6. a
7. i
8. b

9. d
10. g

Completion

11. theories of personality
12. psychoanalysis
13. psychodynamic
14. ego, id, superego (in any order)
15. defense mechanisms
16. oral, anal, phallic (or Oedipal), latency, genital
17. unconscious
18. tested
19. behavioral patterns
20. social-cognitive theories
21. humanist psychologists
22. trait theorists
23. possible selves; ideal, real (in any order)

True-False

24. F
25. T
26. F
27. T

28. T
29. F
30. F
31. T

32. T
33. F
34. F

Self-Test

[Page numbers refer to the Wade and Tavris text.]

1. c (Objective 1; page 457; video program)
2. b (Objective 1; page 457; video program)
3. c (Objective 2; pages 476–477; video program)
4. c (Objective 2; page 478)
5. b (Objective 2; page 477; video program)
6. b (Objective 3; page 479)
7. c (Objective 4; page 481; video program)
8. a (Objective 5; page 485)
9. b (Objective 5; page 486)
10. c (Objective 6; pages 464–465)
11. d (Objective 6; pages 466–467)
12. b (Objective 7; pages 487–489; video program)
13. c (Objective 7; page 488)
14. c (Objective 8; page 459)
15. d (Objective 8; pages 459–461)
16. d (Objective 9; page 464)
17. b (Objective 9; page 462)
18. b (Objective 10; page 489)
19. c (Objective 10; page 489)

Lesson 15   Measuring and Explaining Human Diversity

Review Exercises

Vocabulary Check

1. l
2. f
3. n
4. i
5. c

6. m
7. h
8. o
9. b
10. d

11. g
12. j
13. a
14. e
15. k

Completion

16. reliability, validity, standardization
17. abstractly, learn and profit
18. achievement, aptitude
19. bell-shaped
20. inventories, projective, Rorschach Inkblot Test
21. nature-nurture, identical, methodological
22. education, socioeconomic background (in any order)

True-False

23. F
24. F
25. T
26. T

27. F
28. T
29. F
30. F

31. F
32. T
33. T

Self-Test

[Page numbers refer to the Wade and Tavris text.]

1. a (Objective 1; pages 41–42)
2. c (Objective 1; page 41)
3. b (Objective 2; page 324; video program)
4. d (Objective 2; pages 330–331; video program)
5. b (Objective 2; pages 330–333; video program)
6. b (Objective 3; page 325; video program)
7. c (Objective 3; pages 328–329; video program)
8. d (Objective 4; pages 89, A-6)
9. d (Objective 4; pages 89, A-6)
10. b (Objective 5; video program)
11. c (Objective 5; page 327; video program)
12. a (Objective 6; page 41)
13. b (Objective 6; page 483)
14. b (Objective 7; pages 41, 484; video program)
15. b (Objective 7; pages 91–92)
16. b (Objective 7; pages 91–92)
17. d (Objective 8; video program)
18. a (Objective 8; page 92)
19. d (Objective 9; video program)
20. a (Objective 9; page 329; video program)
21. b (Objective 9; page 333; video program)

Lesson 16　　Child Development

Review Exercises

Vocabulary Check

1. n	6. e	11. h
2. d	7. i	12. m
3. c	8. g	13. j
4. a	9. k	14. f
5. l	10. b	

Completion

15. cognitive, moral, physical, social (in any order)
16. alcohol, cigarettes, German measles (rubella), sexually transmitted diseases (in any order)
17. grasping, sucking (in any order)
18. adaptation, organization (in any order)
19. sensorimotor, object permanence
20. speeding up
21. preoperational, concrete operational
22. contact comfort
23. gender typing, gender identity

True-False

24. F	28. F	32. T
25. T	29. F	33. F
26. F	30. T	
27. T	31. F	

Self-Test

[Page numbers refer to the Wade and Tavris text.]

1. a (Objective 1; page 498)
2. d (Objective 1; page 498)
3. b (Objective 2; page 499)
4. d (Objective 2; pages 499–500)
5. b (Objective 3; page 500)
6. c (Objective 3; page 501)
7. c (Objective 3; page 501)
8. b (Objective 4; pages 506–507; video program)
9. d (Objective 4; page 505)
10. a (Objective 5; page 506; video program)
11. b (Objective 5; page 506; video program)
12. d (Objective 5; page 507; video program)
13. b (Objective 6; pages 508–509; video program)
14. d (Objective 6; video program)
15. b (Objective 6; page 508)
16. c (Objective 6; video program)
17. a (Objective 7; page 502)
18. c (Objective 7; video program)
19. b (Objective 8; page 513)
20. a (Objective 8; pages 513–514)

Lesson 17   Later Childhood and Adolescence

Review Exercises

Vocabulary Check

1. k
2. c
3. e
4. h

5. b
6. i
7. j
8. a

9. d
10. g
11. f

Completion

12. induction, power-assertion
13. behaving in considerate and responsible ways, cognitive ability to evaluate moral dilemmas, empathy for others, the inner voice of conscience (in any order)
14. preconventional morality
15. verbal
16. anxiety and depression, drug abuse and delinquency, social inadequacy (in any order)
17. nocturnal emissions; testes, scrotum, and penis
18. formal operational thought
19. death of a close relative, parental divorce, serious illness (in any order)
20. resilience

True-False

21. F
22. T
23. F

24. F
25. F
26. T

27. F
28. T
29. F

Self-Test

[Page numbers refer to the Wade and Tavris text.]

1. b (Objective 1; page 518)
2. c (Objective 1; page 518)
3. d (Objective 2; pages 511–512)
4. a (Objective 2; page 512)
5. a (Objective 3; pages 511–512)
6. c (Objective 3; page 538)
7. b (Objective 3; page 538)
8. a (Objective 4; pages 523–524)
9. b (Objective 4; page 525; video program)
10. c (Objective 4; page 524; video program)
11. b (Objective 5; pages 507–508; video program)
12. d (Objective 5; pages 507–508; video program)
13. c (Objective 6; page 525)
14. d (Objective 6; page 525)

Lesson 18   Adulthood and Aging

Review Exercises

Vocabulary Check

1. g
2. f
3. d

4. a
5. h
6. b

7. e
8. c
9. i

Completion

10. gerontology
11. psychosocial development; biological drives, societal demands (in any order)
12. divorce, getting married, having children (in any order)
13. basic personality
14. crisis, transition

True-False

15 F
16. T
17. F

18. F
19. T
20. T

21. T

Self-Test

[Page numbers refer to the Wade and Tavris text.]

1. c (Objective 1; telecourse student guide, page 265)
2. d (Objective 1; page 535; telecourse student guide, page 265)
3. c (Objective 2; page 533)
4. d (Objective 2; page 534)
5. b (Objective 2; video program)
6. c (Objective 3; video program)
7. b (Objective 3; page 530; video program)
8. c (Objective 3; pages 530–531; video program)
9. a (Objective 4; pages 532–533; video program)
10. b (Objective 4; page 532; video program)
11. c (Objective 4; page 532; video program)
12. b (Objective 5; pages 274–275)
13. d (Objective 5; pages 274–275)
14. c (Objective 5; pages 274–275)
15. b (Objective 6; pages 532–533; video program)
16. c (Objective 6; pages 532–533; video program)
17. a (Objective 6; video program)

Lesson 19   Health, Stress, and Coping

Review Exercises

Vocabulary Check

1. g
2. f
3. c
4. k
5. d

6. i
7. j
8. n
9. l
10. h

11. a
12. m
13. b
14. e

Completion

15. body's, stressors
16. biological
17. psychoneuroimmunology
18. death of a loved one, daily hassles
19. rethinking, solving (in any order); learning to live with
20. emotional inhibition
21. hostility
22. internal, external
23. no effect, helped reduce
24. "psychologizing"

True-False

25. T
26. F
27. F

28. T
29. T
30. F

31. T
32. T
33. F

Self-Test

[Page numbers refer to the Wade and Tavris text.]

1. a (Objective 1; page 546; video program)
2. c (Objective 2; page 550)
3. d (Objective 2; pages 550–551)
4. c (Objective 3; page 549; video program)
5. b (Objective 3; page 552)
6. c (Objective 4; page 548)
7. d (Objective 4; pages 547–548; video program)
8. a (Objective 5; page 562)
9. c (Objective 5; pages 563–564)
10. b (Objective 6; pages 552–556)
11. d (Objective 6; page 558)
12. b (Objective 7; page 558)
13. c (Objective 7; page 559)
14. b (Objective 8; pages 565–566)
15. a (Objective 8; page 567)
16. d (Objective 9; page 555)
17. d (Objective 9; page 570)

Lesson 20   Psychological Disorders I

Review Exercises

Vocabulary Check

1. e	6. d	11. g
2. i	7. b	12. m
3. a	8. j	13. n
4. c	9. k	14. f
5. o	10. l	15. h

Completion

16. emotional distress, maladaptive behavior, statistical deviation, violation of cultural standards (in any order)

17. descriptive

18. difficulty concentrating, irritability, restlessness, sleep disruption (in any order)

19. manic-depressive

20. brain chemistry, genetic factors (in any order)

21. narcissistic, paranoid (in any order)

22. empathy

True-False

23. F	26. T	29. T
24. F	27. T	
25. F	28. T	

Self-Test

[Page numbers refer to the Wade and Tavris text.]

1. c (Objective 1; pages 576–577; video program)
2. d (Objective 1; page 577)
3. b (Objective 2; page 577; video program)
4. a (Objective 2; page 579)
5. d (Objective 2; pages 578–579)
6. b (Objective 3; page 582; video program)
7. c (Objective 3; page 583)
8. b (Objective 3; page 585)
9. a (Objective 4; page 586)
10. c (Objective 4; page 586)
11. b (Objective 4; page 587)
12. d (Objective 5; pages 587–588; video program)
13. c (Objective 5; page 587)
14. a (Objective 6; page 591)
15. b (Objective 6; page 591)
16. b (Objective 6; page 592)

Lesson 21   Psychological Disorders II

Review Exercises

Vocabulary Check

1. i	5. e	9. a
2. b	6. c	10. g
3. j	7. h	11. l
4. d	8. k	12. f

Completion

13. amnesia, psychogenic
14. dissociative identity disorder (multiple personality disorder)
15. somatoform; conversion disorder, hypochondria (in any order)
16. abuse, use (in any order)
17. disease, tolerance
18. schizophrenia
19. cancer
20. brain
21. organic brain disorders
22. "suicidal types," take all suicide threats seriously

True-False

23. T	27. T	31. F
24. T	28. T	32. F
25. F	29. F	
26. T	30. F	

Self-Test

[Page numbers refer to the Wade and Tavris text.]

1. c (Objective 1; page 595)
2. d (Objective 1; page 596)
3. d (Objective 2; page 578)
4. b (Objective 2; page 578)
5. b (Objective 2; page 578)
6. b (Objective 3; page 599)
7. b (Objective 3; page 600)
8. c (Objective 3; page 604)
9. c (Objective 4; pages 605–606; video program)
10. b (Objective 4; page 607; video program)
11. d (Objective 4; page 606; video program)
12. c (Objective 4; video program)
13. d (Objective 5; pages 607–610; video program)
14. b (Objective 5; pages 608–609; video program)
15. c (Objective 6; video program)
16. a (Objective 6; video program)
17. b (Objective 7; pages 611–612)
18. c (Objective 7; pages 611–612)

Lesson 22   Approaches to Therapy I

Review Exercises

Vocabulary Check

1. e	6. b	11. f
2. a	7. l	12. i
3. h	8. c	13. j
4. m	9. k	
5. g	10. d	

Completion

14. medical treatments, psychotherapy, self-help and community alternatives (in any order)
15. medical, psychological
16. antipsychotic drugs (major tranquilizers)
17. "therapeutic window"
18. psychosurgery
19. psychoanalysis, insight
20. attitudes, behavior (in any order)
21. aversive conditioning, contracts, flooding, systematic desensitization (in any order)
22. client-centered
23. fees

True-False

24. F	28. T	32. T
25. F	29. F	33. F
26. T	30. F	34. T
27. T	31. T	

Self-Test

[Page numbers refer to the Wade and Tavris text.]

1. b (Objective 1; page 617)
2. b (Objective 2; pages 618)
3. d (Objective 2; page 618)
4. d (Objective 3; page 619)
5. d (Objective 3; pages 619–620)
6. c (Objective 3; page 621)
7. b (Objective 3; page 619)
8. c (Objective 4; pages 622–623)
9. b (Objective 4; page 623)
10. b (Objective 5; page 624; video program)
11. a (Objective 5; pages 625)
12. b (Objective 6; pages 625–627)
13. d (Objective 6; page 627; video program)
14. c (Objective 6; page 628)
15. a (Objective 7; page 628; video program)
16. b (Objective 7; page 632; video program)
17. b (Objective 7; page 629)
18. a (Objective 8; page 646; video program)
19. d (Objective 8; page 647; video program)

Lesson 23   Approaches to Therapy II

Review Exercises

Vocabulary Check

1. g
2. b
3. f

4. c
5. d
6. e

7. a

Completion

8. family
9. community programs, self-help and support groups (in any order)
10. therapy, self-help revolution
11. civil-rights, patients'-rights (in any order)
12. group
13. deterioration, dependency
14. myths

True-False

15. T
16. T
17. F

18. F
19. T
20. T

21. F
22. T
23. T

Self-Test

[Page numbers refer to the Wade and Tavris text.]

1. c (Objective 1; page 630; video program)
2. c (Objective 1; page 631; video program)
3. d (Objective 1; pages 629–630)
4. c (Objective 2; page 643)
5. d (Objective 2; page 644; video program)
6. a (Objective 3; page 642)
7. b (Objective 3; page 642)
8. d (Objective 4; page 635)
9. b (Objective 4; page 635)
10. c (Objective 4; page 636)
11. d (Objective 4; pages 636–637)
12. b (Objective 5; pages 625–627)
13. b (Objective 5; page 639)
14. b (Objective 5; page 638)
15. d (Objective 6; pages 640–641)
16. d (Objective 6; page 641)
17. c (Objective 7; page 646)
18. b (Objective 7; page 646)

Lesson 24   Social Psychology

Review Exercises

Vocabulary Check

1. i	5. c	9. g
2. l	6. d	10. a
3. b	7. h	11. e
4. f	8. k	12. j

Completion

13. social psychology; groups, norms, roles (in any order)
14. position, rules
15. "prison study"; guards, prisoners (in any order)
16. situational, dispositional
17. underestimate, accentuate
18. consistency
19. psychological benefit

True-False

20. T	23. T	26. F
21. F	24. F	
22. T	25. F	

Self-Test

[Page numbers refer to the Wade and Tavris text.]

1. a (Objective 1; page 264)
2. c (Objective 1; pages 263–264)
3. d (Objective 2; page 264)
4. c (Objective 2; page 264)
5. d (Objective 3; pages 268–269; video program)
6. b (Objective 3; pages 266–267)
7. a (Objective 3; page 269)
8. a (Objective 4; pages 272–273; video program)
9. b (Objective 4; page 273; video program)
10. d (Objective 4; page 274)
11. c (Objective 5; page 289; video program)
12. c (Objective 5; page 290)
13. d (Objective 5; page 290)
14. a (Objective 5; page 290; video program)
15. c (Objective 6; page 275)
16. b (Objective 6; page 275)
17. b (Objective 7; page 291; video program)
18. d (Objective 7; pages 291–295; video program)
19. d (Objective 7; pages 291–295; video program)

Lesson 25   Individuals and Groups

Review Exercises

Vocabulary Check

1. b
2. d
3. c
4. i

5. j
6. g
7. a
8. h

9. e
10. f

Completion

11. deny, embrace
12. the desire for personal gain, the desire to be accurate, embarrassment, identification with the group, the wish to be liked (in any order)
13. embarrassment, entrapment, lacking a language of protest
14. average
15. groupthink
16. social loafing
17. attitudes, group relations, personality (in any order)
18. socialize informally
19. competition, conformity, deindividuation, roles (in any order)

True-False

20. T
21. T
22. T

23. T
24. T
25. T

26. F
27. F

Self-Test

[Page numbers refer to the Wade and Tavris text.]

1. c (Objective 1; page 270; video program)
2. b (Objective 1; pages 264, 280; video program)
3. d (Objective 2; page 280; video program)
4. b (Objective 2; pages 279–280; video program)
5. c (Objective 2; page 280; video program)
6. a (Objective 3; page 271; video program)
7. c (Objective 3; page 271)
8. a (Objective 4; page 281)
9. b (Objective 5; pages 281–282)
10. c (Objective 5; page 281)
11. a (Objective 6; page 283)
12. b (Objective 6; page 285)
13. c (Objective 7; page 289; video program)
14. d (Objective 7; pages 288–289; video program)
15. b (Objective 8; page 297)
16. a (Objective 8; pages 297–298)
17. b (Objective 9; page 299)

Lesson 26   Issues in Psychology

Review Exercises

Completion

1. biological influences, cognitive influences, learning influences, psychodynamic influences, social and cultural influences (in any order)

2. coping with interpersonal relations, dealing with job stress (in any order)

3. scientific, pop psychology

4. reevaluation of existing theories, research (in any order)

True-False

5. F
6. F
7. F
8. F

Self-Test

[Page numbers refer to the Wade and Tavris text.]

1. b (Objective 1; page 651)

2. d (Objective 1; page 651)

3. b (Objective 2; page 652)

4. c (Objective 3; pages 652–653)

5. a (Objective 4; page 654; video program)

Psychology: The Study of Human Behavior—Quick Reference Guide

Lesson	Telecourse Guide Lesson Title	Textbook Reading Assignment	Television Program
1	What Is Psychology?	Chapter 1, "What Is Psychology?"	What Is Psychology?
2	How Psychologists Know What They Know	Chapter 2, "How Psychologists Know What They Know"	Research Methods
3	The Biology of Behavior	Chapter 4, "Neurons, Hormones, and the Brain," pages 99–112, 133–134	The Biology of Behavior
4	The Brain-Mind Connection	Chapter 4, "Neurons, Hormones, and the Brain," pages 113–133	The Brain-Mind Connection
5	Body Rhythms and Mental States	Chapter 5, "Body Rhythms and Mental States"	Sleep and Dreaming
6	Sensation and Perception	Chapter 6, "Sensation and Perception"	Sensation and Perception
7	Learning	Chapter 7, "Learning and Conditioning"	Learning
8	Memory	Chapter 10, "Memory"	Memory
9	Decision Making and Problem Solving	Chapter 9, "Thinking and Intelligence" pages 305–324, 330–331, and 341	Decision Making and Problem Solving
10	Language	Chapter 3, "Evolution, Genes, and Behavior," pages 72–76; Chapter 9, "Thinking and Intelligence," pages 336–340; and Chapter 14, "Development over the Life Span," pages 504–505	Language
11	Emotion	Chapter 11, "Emotion"	Emotion
12	Motivation	Chapter 12, "Motivation," pages 421–422, 441–452; Chapter 13, "Theories of Personality," pages 467–470, 472–475; Chapter 3, "Evolution, Genes, and Behavior," pages 70–71, 84–89; Chapter 9, "Thinking and Intelligence," pages 321–323, 341; and Chapter 8, "Behavior in Social and Cultural Context," pages 272–274	Motivation
13	Gender and Relationships	Chapter 12, "Motivation," pages 422–423, 426–440; Chapter 14, "Development over the Life Span," pages 513–517; and Chapter 3, "Evolution, Genes, and Behavior," pages 65, 77–80	Gender and Relationships

Psychology: The Study of Human Behavior—Quick Reference Guide

Lesson	Telecourse Guide Lesson Title	Textbook Reading Assignment	Television Program
14	Theories of the Person and Personality	Chapter 13, "Theories of Personality," pages 457–467, 475–482, and 485–492	Personality
15	Measuring and Explaining Human Diversity	Chapter 2, "How Psychologists Do Research," pages 41–42; Chapter 3, "Evolution, Genes, and Behavior," pages 65–68, 80–83, and 89–94; and Chapter 9, "Thinking and Intelligence," pages 324–335. Also review Chapter 13, "Theories of Personality," pages 483–486, and Appendix, "Statistical Methods," pages A-4 to A-6	Intelligence
16	Child Development	Chapter 14, "Development over the Life Span," pages 497–504, 505–510, and 513–517, and Chapter 12, "Motivation," pages 422–425	Cognitive Development
17	Later Childhood and Adolescence	Chapter 14, "Development over the Life Span," pages 510–512, 518–527, and 537–538, and review pages 505–509	Adolescent Development
18	Adulthood and Aging	Chapter 14, "Development over the Life Span," pages 529–537, and Chapter 8, "Behavior in Social and Cultural Context," pages 274–275	Adult Development
19	Health, Stress, and Coping	Chapter 15, "Health, Stress, and Coping"	Health, Stress, and Coping
20	Psychological Disorders I	Chapter 16, "Psychological Disorders," pages 575–594	What Is Normal?
21	Psychological Disorders II	Chapter 16, "Psychological Disorders," pages 578, 595–611	Psychotic Disorders
22	Approaches to Therapy I	Chapter 17, "Approaches to Treatment and Therapy," pages 617–629 and 646	Approaches to Therapy
23	Approaches to Therapy II	Chapter 17, "Approaches to Treatment and Therapy," pages 625–646	Therapy Choices
24	Social Psychology	Chapter 8, "Behavior in Social and Cultural Context," pages 263–278, 288–301	Social Psychology
25	Individuals and Groups	Chapter 8, "Behavior in Social and Cultural Context," pages 279–288, 296–301, and review pages 266–268	Conformity, Obedience, and Dissent
26	Issues in Psychology	Epilogue, "Taking Psychology with You"	Issues in Psychology